PLANTS THAT HEAL

Essays On Botanical Medicine

David Crow, L.Ac.

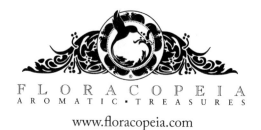

FLORACOPEIA
AROMATIC · TREASURES

www.floracopeia.com

Table of Contents

Acknowledgments

These essays were written between 2003 and 2013, primarily as papers that were presented at the Medicines From the Earth and Southwest Conference On Botanical Medicine symposiums. Collectively, they outline a broad vision of how medicinal plants can be used for healing the individual, society and environment, ranging from specific uses of herbs and essential oils, to the grassroots healthcare offered by community gardens, to how plants continually purify and regenerate the biosphere.

Many thanks are due to Linnea and Larry Wardwell, for the invitations to participate in their renowned and popular herbal conferences. Many thanks are also due to the National Ayurvedic Medical Association for its invitations to teach many times at their conferences, culminating last year with the invitation to give the opening keynote address.

David Crow, L.Ac.

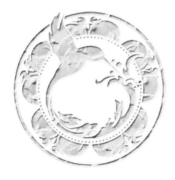

I

The People's Pharmacy
Creating Grassroots Healthcare Systems

Introduction

The last century brought immense improvements in health and longevity to people in the US. Some of these benefits can be attributed to medical advances, but most were the result of better sanitation, nutrition, and overall quality of life. Now, many of the improvements that were gained are being lost, and new threats to individual and collective health are emerging. Instead of open sewers, we have ubiquitous environmental contamination; instead of malnutrition from inadequate intake of food, we have widespread nutrition-related illnesses caused by degradation of the food chain. While modern medicine has made great advances, iatrogenic illnesses are among the leading causes of morbidity and fatality, and preventable and treatable chronic degenerative diseases have reached epidemic levels.

The Root Causes of Illness

Most health problems in modern America can be attributed to five root causes. These are:

Nutrition
Environmental pollution
Socio economic stresses
Spiritual emptiness
Medical treatments and drug toxicity

Holistic medical systems, including Traditional Chinese Medicine, Ayurveda, and Naturopathic medicine, offer significant benefits in the treatment of symptoms arising from these root causes, especially those related to nutrition, environmental toxins, and iatrogenic illness. Every clinician, however, is well acquainted with the limitations of what natural medicine can do when these root causes are not adequately resolved in a patient's life.

Over the years, my clinical work has evolved toward an increasingly personalized form of practice, which strives to uncover, understand, and remove the root causes of illness, while simultaneously treating its symptoms. As a result, I have become aware of the urgent need for a new form of medicine, one which raises the overall level of environmental, social, nutritional, and spiritual well-being. It would not be "alternative," "complementary," or "integrated" medicine, although it could be used in many cases as an alternative or complementary therapy, or integrated with other healthcare modalities. Rather, it would be a parallel system of medicine—grassroots, community-supported, cost-effective, plant-based healthcare, accessible to everyone. In other words, folk medicine: using medicinal and nutritive plants grown in our neighborhoods, according to common knowledge passed down within families and communities.

Community-Supported Plant-Based Healthcare

The revival of folk medicine and the creation of community-supported plant-based healthcare depends on many types of social, botanical, educational, and environmental projects and participants working together, including:

- Community and urban gardens
- School gardens
- Eco-villages
- Eco-preserves
- Agro-forests
- Nurseries and small herb farms
- Botanical gardens
- Seed banks
- Practitioners and educators of herbal medicine

Community and urban gardens

Community gardens and urban gardening have a long history, and are now re-emerging as viable alternatives to both modern agribusiness and destructive traditional farming methods such as slash and burn. Community gardens come in all shapes and sizes: from tiny, inner city plots tended by homeless people, to entire neighborhoods planted with foods and medicines. These gardens can be as simple as potted plants on balconies and rooftops, and as innovative as edible parks. In developing countries, urban and community gardens are a primary source of nutrition and income for countless families.

Community gardens are the foundation of grassroots healthcare. Without a strong nutritional foundation from affordable, locally grown organic foods, it is difficult to improve the standards of health in society. When medicinal plants and foods are cultivated together, folk medicine becomes part of the community.

When neighborhoods are transformed into gardens, numerous social problems are resolved: crime decreases, community and family bonds are strengthened. Gardens are places of beauty and spiritual solace, which bring happiness to those suffering from stress and emotional difficulties. Prison gardens, for example, are now recognized as one of the best paths to genuine criminal rehabilitation. By transforming our cities into living pharmacies and sources of nourishment, the five root causes of sickness can all be alleviated.

School gardens

School gardens are a rapidly developing aspect of community and urban gardening. In outdoor classrooms students find more enjoyment in learning; thus attention difficulties and behavior problems are reduced. Emotional growth and social skills are enhanced when students observe the processes of nature at work and are given responsibility for caretaking plants and animals. The high quality nutrition provided by the gardens, along with the physical activity of gardening, improves the overall health of students and teachers alike.

School gardens are the seeds for a sustainable plant-based culture. Many of the academic studies that are encouraged in today's schools will become obsolete in the coming years, and many new fields will become important parts of public education, including organic gardening, natural medicine, permaculture, sustainable ecology, alternative energy, and non-toxic industries. As more students begin careers in these areas, society will be positively transformed.

Eco-preserves, agro-forests, botanical gardens, and seed banks

Extinction of plant and animal species is accelerating. It is estimated that 34,000 species of plants are currently facing extinction, including many important sources of food, medicine, fiber, oil, and fuel. There are only two solutions to this global problem: the preservation of existing habitats, and widespread cultivation of endangered plants. At this time, only a relatively small number of medicinal plants are in sustainable cultivation; the majority continue to be overharvested from dwindling wild sources.

Eco-preserves, agro-forests, botanical gardens, and seed banks are playing a critical role in caretaking the genetic base of the plant realm for future generations. As community gardens flourish and folk medicine takes root in more neighborhoods, more plants can be brought into greater cultivation, drawing on the resources preserved by these larger entities. An excellent example is the work of Paul Strauss and the many volunteers at the United Plant Savers Sanctuary, who have renovated a degraded forest area into a world-class botanical preserve for the major endangered medicinal plants of the US. Projects such as these hold the key to the continuation of herbal traditions throughout the world, and the return of medicinal plants to society.

Eco-villages

Eco-villages represent the synthesis of all the elements necessary for the creation of community-supported plant-based healthcare. Eco-villages are based on innovative paradigms of self-sufficiency and independence from the economic and ecological disasters of corporate globalization; grassroots medicine is an important part of this self-sufficiency. Larger eco-villages produce their own food and medicines; some produce medicinal products for income, and some have small clinics operated by trained herbalists. Some are involved in agro-forestry or are linked with eco-preserves. Many offer educational programs in a wide variety of ecological, spiritual, and healthcare topics.

Practitioners and educators of herbal medicine

The last decade has seen an astronomical increase in the use of herbs by the general public, stimulated by the health food and natural products industries, the spread of alternative and complementary therapies, and the urgent need for nontoxic medicine. In order for herbal medicine to be further integrated into society at the grassroots level so that these medicines are available in a cost-effective way for everyone, the knowledge of how to grow and use the plants must once again become part of family traditions. Those who have training and clinical expertise with herbs can play important roles in bringing phytotherapies to a broader level of acceptance and use by society, and in establishing herbal medicine as a viable grassroots healthcare system.

There are several ways that herbalists and other healthcare practitioners can support the revival of community-supported folk medicine. The most important is helping to create and maintain community and urban gardens. When community gardens have the active support and participation of knowledgeable herbalists, information about the propagation, cultivation, harvesting, and use of medicinal plants becomes an ongoing part of the collective learning experience. Another way is to encourage patients to grow their own medicines, specifically those needed for their health conditions. This can easily lead to the creation of a network of gardens in a neighborhood, where a wide variety of herbs are being grown by different people. When herbs are grown in communities, either collectively in community-supported gardens or in a network of neighborhood gardens, many teaching opportunities arise naturally. Hands-on medicine-making classes, horticultural workshops, and classes on the use of specific plants or the treatment of specific health concerns are an excellent way for herbal practitioners to support folk medicine; it is also one of the best ways to build a clinical practice.

The Need For Grassroots Healthcare

The need for grassroots community-supported plant-based healthcare is becoming more urgent. The reasons for this include:

- High cost of healthcare
- Lack of insurance coverage
- Need for affordable nontoxic medicines
- Loss of medicinal plant species
- Loss of ethnobotanical knowledge
- Need for fresh, high-quality, locally grown foods and medicines
- Loss of communities and degradation of urban environments

High cost of healthcare and lack of insurance coverage

While having the world's most expensive per capita medical system, the US ranks among the lowest of the developed countries for quality of healthcare. Almost fifty million people now lack any form of health insurance, and an almost equal number are inadequately insured. This combination of high medical costs and lack of basic health coverage is causing impoverishment on top of illness, while the domination of the medical profession by the insurance industry is placing tremendous strain on the integrity and functionality of modern medicine. Although there is an increasing demand for universal healthcare coverage, there is little political will to change the current conditions.

Need for affordable nontoxic medicines

Even if universal coverage became a reality, it would probably cover only the basics of modern allopathic medicine. The great limitation and deficiency of modern allopathic pharmaceutical drugs is their inability to increase immunity, enhance nutritional status, regenerate vitality, restore humoral and energetic homeostasis, or detoxify; in reality, the epidemic of iatrogenic illnesses can be attributed to the adverse effects of drugs on immunity, nutritional status, vitality, homeostasis, and detoxification processes. Only the phyto-nutrients and medicinal constituents of botanical plants can effectively perform these crucial functions. Unfortunately, high quality herbal preparations are becoming increasingly expensive, and many people cannot afford the out-of-pocket expenses necessary to treat chronic conditions.

Loss of medicinal plants

One of the primary reasons for the high cost of many herbal medicines is decreasing supplies of plant materials. Uncontrolled overharvesting has brought numerous important medicinal species to the brink of extinction. As global demand and need for herbal medicines increase, overharvesting accelerates. This depletes natural populations, which increases the value of the plant, which in turn stimulates more overharvesting. Unfortunately, many important medicines will be lost forever due to this destructive cycle, and other plants will become so rare that they will be affordable only as luxury items for the wealthy. The only way that many medicinal and nutritional plant species will be saved from this fate is through widespread cultivation, both as commercial products and in community gardens as folk medicines.

Loss of ethnobotanical knowledge

Medicinal plants, the habitats they come from, and the understanding of their uses are inseparable. As medicinal plants are lost and the habitats they come from vanish, the accumulated knowledge of age-old ethnobotanical traditions also perishes. Community-based healthcare again offers the hope of preserving this valuable heritage. When plants are brought into widespread local cultivation, the knowledge of their cultivation, harvesting, preparation, and use can once again be preserved within families.

Need for high-quality locally grown foods and medicine

Fossil fuels are a finite resource; our modern lifestyle and agricultural methods, which are largely based on fossil fuels, are therefore finite. It is likely that in the near future, instability of oil supplies, worsening economic conditions, and the cumulative hidden costs of destructive agribusiness practices will drive the cost of growing and transporting food higher; the result will be increased malnutrition and decreased immunity in the population. Cultivating foods and medicines in local communities will reduce dependency on agribusiness and fossil fuels, and increase the general level of nutritional status and resistance to illness.

Loss of communities and degradation of urban environments

For many people, urban environments and the stresses of modern culture are the primary sources of sickness and suffering. The current degraded and deteriorating condition of many urban and suburban areas is the result of short-sighted city planning, which has placed cars, business interests, and racial segregation above the interests of people, nature, and health. Unpleasant and unrewarding careers in unhealthy work environments, so common as to be accepted as normal, present a formidable challenge to those seeking to improve their wellbeing.

Cities do not have to be unpleasant, unhealthy, and stressful places to live and work, however. As many projects are proving, cities can be places where business thrives in car-free environments, homeless people grow their own food, smog and pollution are dramatically reduced, opportunities for right livelihood abound, and the general level of nutritional wellbeing is improved through community gardening.

Through the universal human need for plants, plant-based healthcare can be linked to the re-greening of urban environments, resulting in many fundamental improvements in public and environmental health. The collective work of tending community gardens helps restores community and family bonds. Ecological cities create numerous job opportunities in non-toxic industries, which provide alternatives to the stressful disease-causing careers of the modern corporate world. Training homeless people to cultivate organic foods and medicines in urban settings is potentially one of the best solutions to the increasingly serious social problems of urban environmental degradation. By replanting cities, both with community gardens and urban forests, they will become cleaner, quieter, and more beautiful.

Creating Grassroots Healthcare

Building a grassroots movement to grow and utilize medicinal and nutritive plants in a collective manner requires commitment and resources originating from individuals, neighborhoods, and communities. In order for this movement to quickly gain momentum and have long-term success, it must be embraced by city planners, have the cooperation of numerous professions and organizations, and receive funding from governments. While this seems unlikely under the current political climate, worsening environmental, social, and medical conditions are bringing about significant changes in cultural priorities. Historically, the more economies suffer, the more people work together at the grassroots level to provide for their needs. A striking example of this is Cuba: in response to economic and political isolation, it has become a leading model of self-sufficient urban gardening and government-sponsored, community-supported folk medicine.

Numerous models of sustainable community-based healthcare are well established throughout the world. These projects comprise a network of various functions related to the preservation, propagation, and utilization of medicinal plants, and are therefore crucial for the building of a grassroots movement as the greater global need increases. When social, medical, and environmental priorities change, when political will is activated, and when government support becomes a reality, these projects will be the repositories of plants and knowledge from which sustainable cultures can be created.

II

Farm to Pharmacy

Introduction

Farm to Pharmacy is the inspiration of William Siff, an acupuncturist, herbalist and owner of the Goldthread Farm and Apothecary in Northampton, Massachusetts. Now in its third year, this unique and innovative educational program introduces students to the full spectrum of herbal medicine, from cultivation of plants to their use in clinical practice, with an emphasis on creating a sustainable, non-toxic, and cost-effective community-based healthcare system. This article gives a basic overview of the program, what has been accomplished so far, the questions and challenges that have come with such an endeavor, and the goals and benefits that we hope to achieve in the coming years.

Background

The Farm to Pharmacy programs take place from April through October at Goldthread Herb Farm and Apothecary in the foothills of the Berkshires in western Massachusetts. There are currently three simultaneous levels of trainings: a seven-month residential training; three week-long intensives offered during the spring, summer and fall; and a summer program for children. Additionally, a two-year residential program is being launched in the spring of 2012. William teaches all the programs, and I co-teach with him during the seasonal intensives.

In both the seven-month internship and the seasonal intensives, students begin in the greenhouse, tending to seedlings and learning the fundamentals of propagating over one hundred species of medicinal plants. As the season progresses students learn plant identification, soil health and composition, composting strategies, maintenance and design of educational and production gardens, and harvesting and processing techniques. A special part of the program is the unique opportunity to participate in the distillation of essential oils and hydrosols over a wood fire in an eighty-five gallon commercial still, including conifer oils wild-harvested from the surrounding forests and selected crops such as lavender and yarrow grown on the farm.

As the weeks progress students begin learning the skills necessary to be a community herbalist. Utilizing various preparations for their own health needs, students gain a deep experiential understanding of the healing qualities of medicinal plants within their own bodies. The physiological actions of herbs as well as basic chemistry are taught within the context of traditional Western, Chinese, and Ayurvedic medical systems. The preparation of tinctures, syrups, elixirs, teas, salves, and oils are all introduced.

In the final phase of the program students work under the guidance of a licensed healthcare professional to learn the clinical uses of the herbs they have grown for common illnesses.

This educational approach combines working with living herbs in the soil, studying the academic and scientific knowledge of phytomedicine and then utilizing finished herbal products for practical healing purposes; in this way students gain a truly holistic understanding of the power of plants.

Objectives

The stated objective of the programs is "to provide participants with the practical skills, medical knowledge and confidence to integrate herbal medicine into the lives of their families and communities according to their personal aspirations. The program is ideal for teachers interested in integrating herbal medicine into their curriculum in school gardens, or herbalists and practitioners of natural medicine who would like to deepen their connection to the plants and increase their understanding of herbal theory. Farmers can take what they learn and integrate it into their existing agricultural projects, and community activists will gain the tools necessary to apply herbal medicine to areas of social justice, urban renewal, and healthcare reform."

As the programs have evolved, these objectives have become more developed, and new ones have also emerged. These include:

Developing parameters of what constitutes safe and effective folk medicine practiced by families and individuals without professional licenses.

Developing a curriculum for grassroots healthcare education that can be easily duplicated in every community.

Developing a model of a simple herbal garden that provides a basis for a home pharmacy.

Training people how to distill essential oils from locally available plants for high potency medicines.

Integration of medicinal plants into local farms, farmers markets and Community Supported Agriculture (CSA's), and the creation of Community Supported Medicine modeled on the CSA system.

Developing the role of the traditional apothecary as the interface between communities, herb farms, holistic licensed practitioners, school systems, community gardens and other groups.

A Simple Home Herbal Garden

The foundation of the Farm to Pharmacy training program is a group of about forty species of medicinal plants. The criteria that we used for choosing these herbs were:

1. Can be grown easily in most locations in the US.
2. Provide a wide range of medicinal functions and therapeutic benefits.
3. Safe for general usage without concern for acute or chronic toxicity.

The garden has five main categories of herbs.

Aromatic culinary herbs: Oreganos, thymes, marjorams, sages, basils, rosemary, fennel, garlic

Herbaceous garden medicinals: Catnip, lavenders, mints, chamomiles, lemon balm, motherwort, skullcap, St. Johnswort, calendula, California poppy, arnica

Weedy plants tending to grow wild: Yarrow, plantain, nettles, dandelion, mullein, raspberry

Medicinal roots: Ashwaghanda, asparagus, astragalus, elecampane, angelica, marshmallow, comfrey, echinacea, burdock, valerian

Other species: Aloe vera, elderberry

Our intention in creating this list was to have a template that can be easily duplicated for every home anywhere in the country, even if the garden is only grown in pots in the kitchen or on the porch. Our hope is that a simple undertaking such as this can produce significant nutritional and immunological benefits at a grassroots level, by introducing a wider range of plant species into the daily diet as well as educating people in the lost knowledge of how to care for themselves using safe and pleasant remedies that were once part of every home.

Home Pharmacy

In addition to training and encouraging people to start small medicinal gardens, another primary objective is showing people how to create and use a simple home pharmacy. The system that we developed is based on placing different forms of herbal medicines in different parts of the home, to create a kind of "herbal lifestyle." These remedies are based on the primary list of herbs in the home garden, but include other important and easily available species as well.

Kitchen medicine: spice collection and fresh herbs from the garden used in cooking and teas; collection of dried herbs for teas; tonic roots for soups

Dining room: herbal bitters and digestive herbs to accompany meals

Medicine cabinet: stronger tinctures and essential oils for specific medical needs as colds and flus; first aid remedies, salves, etc

Bath: oils, salts and herbal preparations

Bedroom: herbs and essential oils for relaxation, sleep, sensuality and intimacy

Additionally, the home pharmacy also includes a small collection of the most important essential oils. The criteria for these oils are that they are easily available, affordable, effective for a wide range of common conditions, and low potential for toxicity. These are: lavender, helichrysum, tea tree, eucalyptus and/or conifer oils, jatamansi (spikenard), and frankincense and/or palo santo.

Distillation of Essential Oils

One of the unique aspects of the Farm to Pharmacy program is the distillation of essential oils from fresh harvested and wild-crafted aromatic plants. Students participate in the entire process over the course of a full day, from gathering of the plant material, its preparation, setting up and firing the still, observing the stages of distillation and separation of the oil from hydrosol. The end result is not only an in-depth introduction to this ancient art and science and an extraordinary olfactory experience, but a great appreciation for how much biomass, time and labor is distilled into a small vial of valuable oil.

The preparation for distillation takes place during the day, and the still is fired over a wood fire in the early evening. For many students, this is the high point of the program, as it becomes far more than just an aromatherapy class: with a full moon rising, fireflies in the trees and excellent companions, it is a magical time of watching the slow alchemical transformation of botanical life force and pondering the mysteries of nature.

From the perspective of grassroots healthcare, this is possibly the pinnacle of folk medicine, as the production of essential oils and hydrosols elevates herbal medicines to a pharmaceutical level of potency, more so than other extracting methods. This simple technology is a literal and symbolic form of medical empowerment for communities, as it gives the ability to transform plants into their most concentrated form, now widely recognized as agents that have the power to destroy microbial pathogens that have become resistant to modern antibiotics.

Grassroots Healthcare: Defining Four Levels of Medical Practice

Like other herbal education programs that do not lead to licensure, one of the first challenges to offering the Farm to Pharmacy training was to define the scope of practice of folk medicine. We were aware early on that we did not want our students returning to their communities and undertaking to treat conditions they were not qualified to treat, but we also knew that people would be seeking out their advice and assistance for medical problems.

Our political view is that access to medicinal plants and the knowledge of their uses are the right of every person in society, and our goal is to support a revival of folk medicine which empowers individuals and families to care for themselves. Yet the reality is that the dominant insurance-driven pharmaceutical-based healthcare system has created an immense burden on society by excessively and unnecessarily medicating people for simple conditions that are easily treated with folk medicine on the one hand and on the other by leaving people no option but to pay out of pocket for complementary and alternative treatments. Furthermore, this dominance has also led to a situation where patients are confronted on the one hand by the failures of pharmaceuticals, such as MRSA and drug toxicity, and on the other hand by active resistance to natural alternatives by the medical industry.

The result is the absence of a knowledge base for self-care and treatment, that is so basic it is not unrealistic to say that modernized developed society is probably the first time in human history when people have largely forgotten what real food is and how to cure themselves of common ailments. The result is that people embrace toxic medication when it is not needed and at the same time have wildly unrealistic expectations, both negative and positive, about what herbal medicines can and cannot do.

In order to address these complex questions, we developed a simplistic yet medically accurate system to help our students, some of whom bring challenging health issues to the program, to understand what constitutes the ethical and legal parameters of "grassroots healthcare." This system is based on the recognition that there are four distinct types of practice, which have become confused and distorted due to the dominance of allopathic medicine and loss of herbal traditions. These four levels are:

Grassroots Healthcare

This level can be defined by alternate terms such as "folk medicine," "kitchen medicine," and "home pharmacy." This level is basically the use of simple herbal remedies for common and uncomplicated conditions. More specifically, the scope of this practice includes the numerous ways of using herbs that are available to everyone, including culinary herbs, spices and tonic roots in the diet for preventive and curative purposes, essential oils for aromatherapy, dried herbs for teas, tinctures for more controlled dosages of important remedies, and so on.

Licensed Holistic Practitioners

This level is defined as utilizing the knowledge, skills and experience of licensed holistic practitioners, including acupuncturists, naturopaths, chiropractors, and holistic MD's.

Allopathic Medicine

This level of medicine is defined as what most people consider to be the primary scope of practice in the US, that is, allopathic-trained physicians using conventional diagnostic methods and pharmaceutical prescriptions.

Emergency Medicine

This level of medicine is defined as trauma medicine and acute care.

We begin by defining these four levels of practice, and then educating students about what constitutes each level when it comes to common illnesses and diseases that affect each organ system. Some simple examples of this system are:

Respiratory system

Grassroots healthcare: prevention and treatment of common colds and flus using herbal teas, tinctures and essential oils

Holistic practitioner: acupuncture, dietary and herbal programs for treatment of asthma when self-care is insufficient

Allopathic medicine: treatment of acute pulmonary infections such as pneumonia and TB, pharmaceutical management of asthma when necessary

Emergency medicine: acute asthma attack

Digestive system

Grassroots healthcare: kitchen medicine to treat common and uncomplicated digestive complaints

Holistic practitioner: acupuncture, dietary and herbal programs for holistic treatment of IBS, colitis, GERD

Allopathic medicine: diagnosis of parasitic conditions, diagnosis and pharmaceutical management of colitis and gastric ulcers when necessary

Emergency medicine: diagnosis and treatment of diverticulitis, appendicitis

What we discovered when we started defining these levels of practice was that the grassroots healthcare component was by far the most important for improving the health of society overall, for several reasons. First, it is the most affordable, cost effective and least toxic for the widest range of common conditions, especially when the home herbal garden is included. Second, it encompasses the herbal and dietary aspects of what most holistic practitioners would prescribe. Third, it is preventive and many times curative for the epidemics of infectious and chronic degenerative diseases that allopathic medicine finds increasingly difficult or impossible to treat. Fourth, it supports immunity and detoxification when allopathic medicine is needed. Fifth, it prevents many types of acute conditions that require emergency medicine and is regenerative after acute care and emergency medicine are needed.

All of these benefits can be summed up as stemming from the ability of medicinal plants to provide nourishment, immune enhancement, regeneration, adaptogenic powers and detoxification.

The Role of Community Apothecaries

In traditional cultures the use of simple herbal remedies was common knowledge; our intention in the Farm to Pharmacy program is to help reestablish some degree of that knowledge, without crossing legal or ethical boundaries of medical practice that are the rightful domain of licensed clinicians. The fundamental challenge in doing this is that essentially, everyone needs plant medicines, and this need will only increase as stresses, toxins, and nutritional deficiencies proliferate and spread. From strong athletes who wish to enhance performance to chemotherapy patients who cannot eat, from new mothers struggling with a chronically ill infant to those needing rejuvenation in old age, there is no condition or phase of life that cannot be benefited or treated with botanical medicines.

Plant medicines and plant-based therapies, therefore, represent not just a different form of treatment in contrast to allopathic pharmaceutical medicine, but a radically different relationship with our bodies, our health, and the celestial, terrestrial and ancestral energies and elements that plants first concentrate in themselves and then transmit to us. Looked at in this way, the loss of herbal traditions is not just the loss of important information about how to use the gifts of the natural world to strengthen and heal ourselves, but the loss of a fundamental biological and spiritual connection to the natural world that has profound implications for the human race.

An apothecary, therefore, should not merely be an outlet for retail products of the herb industry, but a matrix of activities that work to restore society's relationship with plants and the local ecosystems they grow in, while simultaneously addressing the lack of nutritive and preventative healthcare at the community level. A truly holistic apothecary should serve the following purposes:

To encourage and support regional production of medicinal plants as the source of raw materials for locally produced medicines.

To offer locally produced medicines and education about their uses to the community.

To function as a training center for community herbalists.

To offer the clinical and/or consulting services of a trained holistic practitioner who serves as the interface between the folk medicine and the allopathic levels of healthcare.

To launch and support community health projects such as community and school gardens, herb pharmacies in schools and nursing homes.

While it is health concerns that bring people to natural medicines, what they receive when they enter the world of living herbs is something that reaches far beyond substituting a natural pill for a synthetic one. It is, in fact, an aesthetic realm of sensory experiences that reawaken the vitality damaged by the artificiality of our environment. In a fundamental way, we are sick from lack of natural beauty, movement of the body in the outdoors, delicious and strengthening flavors, pleasant aromas of nature, the soothing sounds of water and birds, and the feelings of changing seasons. A holistic apothecary, therefore, serves as a doorway back to those sources of healing, not just by providing medicines from the surrounding countryside but also by drawing people into the wider cultural activities that it represents.

What we are finding in the Farm to Pharmacy programs is that simply by returning to the plants on the farm and in the apothecary, by resuming some semblance of the ancient rhythms of work and rest, by directly tasting and smelling what is not normally in our diets, and by reconnecting the lost threads of what was once one of humanity's major activities, that vitality is renewed and toxic stress is removed, while the herbs become the vehicle for a new way of living.

Community Supported Medicine

One of the most innovative, and in my opinion revolutionary inspirations for the reintroduction of herbal medicine into communities is the offering of locally grown species based on the model of community supported agriculture (CSA). In this system individuals and families purchase shares in local farms, thereby sharing both the risk and the economic investment; in exchange they receive regular allotments of whatever is being produced by the farms as it becomes available during the seasons.

The Goldthread Herb Farm is located in a region that probably has the highest concentration of CSA's in the country, so it was a simple step for William to begin offering shares, not of produce, but of medicinal plants and their preparations to the local communities. Originally, we referred to this as the country's first Herbal CSA, but William has now given the system an official name: Community Supported Medicine, or CSM.

Community Supported Medicine serves several important purposes. First, it creates a direct connection between the producers and the users of medicinal plants, which has a multitude of benefits: increased freshness of medicines, aesthetic appreciation of growing plants in their environment, de-commodification of herbs, strengthening of local economies, and so on. Second, it creates a new level in the four-tiered scheme of healthcare, which is folk medicine guided by a licensed holistic practitioner, thereby strengthening the base of knowledge that was once in families. Third, it addresses the widespread need for greater nutritive diversity in the diet by providing a range of culinary spices and herbal teas for daily use, in addition to the stronger herbal preparations such as tinctures and cough syrups. Fourth, it strengthens and builds community and locality and reduces the need for importation and global commerce, thereby creating the foundation for a post-petroleum society.

Conclusion

Farm to Pharmacy began as an educational program, but has evolved into a multi-faceted approach to transforming healthcare. Taken together, the combination of herbal education, distillation of essential oils, cultivation of home medicinal gardens, home pharmacies, the role of apothecaries and Community Supported Medicine is a complete mandala of interrelated social, medical, economic and ecological functions and objectives that has the capacity to fill the void of knowledge created by our over-dependence on industrialized medicine and elevate botanical medicine to its rightful place at this time of need.

III

Fukushima and Beyond
Research On Herbs For Protection From Radiation

Introduction

Following the nuclear catastrophe at Fukushima many people in the natural health community began discussing the use of herbs for protection against radiation. While the radiation released from that accident is a gravely serious and ongoing environmental health issue, especially for children growing up in the vicinity of the reactors, it is far from the only source of radiotoxicity in the biosphere. A quick perusal of various references reveals some sobering statistics:

Since 1950 there have been twenty-eight civilian nuclear accidents, seven of which are classified as nuclear disasters.

There have been sixty-two reported military nuclear accidents, including warheads dropped, exploded or vanished during airplane accidents, reactor meltdowns, accidents during nuclear testing, fires at weapons factories, sinking of submarines with reactors and warheads, and nuclear powered satellites falling back to earth. (1)

An incomplete list of nuclear reactors used for power, research or military purposes reveals that there are close to 1,000 reactors worldwide. (2)

It is estimated that there have been ninety-nine accidents at nuclear power plants from 1952 to 2009. Fifty-seven accidents have occurred since the Chernobyl disaster, and almost two-thirds (fifty-six out of ninety-nine) of all nuclear-related accidents have occurred in the U.S. (3)

There have been eight military attacks against nuclear reactors.

There have been a total of 2,123 nuclear detonations for "testing" purposes by various countries, including atmospheric, underground, underwater, and in space; the majority of them have been done by the US. (4)

This list could be further lengthened to include the tons of depleted uranium weapons used in Eastern Europe and the Middle East, the leaking of highly radioactive waste into the Columbia River Valley from the military's Hanford site, the use of radioactive materials in consumer products such as home smoke detectors, and so on.

When considering the combined amount and longevity of radioactive elements that have been released into the environment, the meltdown of the reactors at Fukushima appear as only one further addition to a cumulative biospheric poisoning that will span millennia and have profound impacts on all forms of life. Therefore, our relationship to medicinal plants and the protective compounds that they potentially offer should be viewed as a long-term biological necessity.

Personally, I have two views about this subject. The first was influenced by an interview that I did with nuclear activist Dr. Helen Caldecott. I asked her what she thought about the use of environmental remediation technologies and using natural medicine to support health, and whether these approaches had any value. She replied no, that once the radionuclides were in the environment they will find their way into the human body, and once they have started bio-accumulating in the body they will cause damage. In her opinion, the only real answer is prevention.

In an ultimate sense I think Dr. Caldecott's view is correct, as there are limits to what natural medicine can do in the face of rising toxicity levels around us. On the other hand, as an herbalist I know from both study and practice that medicinal plants provide the body with important compounds that support a range of physiological functions that may translate into systemic protection from radiotoxicity including antioxidant, immune enhancing, hepatoprotective, anti-mutagenic and detoxifying.

This paper, therefore, is an overview of various studies that have examined these physiological benefits of some botanical species, and the potential they may hold for protection from radiation, from both environmental contamination and medical treatments. It is offered with both the optimistic view that plants can help us, especially those people whose immune and glandular functions are already developed and strong, and the pragmatic view that as coming generations are exposed to increasingly high levels of cumulative radioactive toxins in the environment that the effectiveness of natural medicine will probably decline.

This decline will be due to exposure to higher levels of radioactivity earlier in life, even in utero, which will weaken and mutate the constitutional and genetic strength of each subsequent generation; at the same time plants, both foods and medicines, will be bio-accumulating radioactive contamination of the soil and water. The accumulation of radiation in medicinal species is already a problem that herbalists should be aware of: exports of green tea have been banned from certain regions of Japan, and contamination of seaweeds along the west coast of the U.S. with cesium from Fukushima has been found.

Radioactive Elements

The terms "radionuclide" and "radioactive isotope" refer to atoms that have unstable nuclei that are undergoing radioactive decay, in the process releasing their excess energy as ionizing radiation. All forms of ionizing radiation cause similar damage at a cellular level, with some being more penetrating than others. The elements we are concerned with are those created from manmade nuclear reactions, rather than naturally occurring such as cosmic rays from the sun; we are specifically concerned about those elements when they contaminate the environment from nuclear detonations or by escaping from reactors, where they bio-accumulate in the food chain and are ingested by eating or breathing them; once in the tissues their ionizing radiation damages cellular DNA.

The easiest way to understand the threat of radiation and the purpose of finding botanical protection from it is this: after several decades of environmental contamination with long-lived radionuclides, all of us now have these elements accumulating in our bodies where they are emitting ionizing radiation into the surrounding cells and tissues.

There are numerous radioactive elements that are released into the environment from nuclear detonations or meltdowns of reactors. Some decay quickly, while others will persist for hundreds or thousands of years or longer. Each of these elements has an affinity to different organs and tissues where it accumulates; for example, Iodine 131 accumulates in the thyroid and is responsible for the high rates of thyroid abnormalities (and presumed later cancers) in children living in the vicinity of Fukushima. The primary radionuclides that Americans were exposed to after Fukushima were Iodine 131, which has a half-life of eight days but was detected traveling worldwide, and Cesium 137 and 134, with half-lives of around thirty years, which were detected over wide areas including the Western United States. Plutonium, the most toxic and long lasting, was released into the environment during the meltdowns as well; there are conflicting reports about how far it has travelled, ranging from a short distance from the reactors to globally. (5)

Radioprotection and Detoxification

Radionuclides cause a number of illnesses, but they are primarily the etiology of various cancers and birth defects. Herbal medicine for protection from radiation would therefore be closely related to protocols for cancer prevention in general.

The subject of radionuclides, their toxicity and longevity, how and where they accumulate in the body and the range of diseases they can cause are beyond the scope of this paper; this report is focused only on presenting a list of botanical species that have been studied for their radioprotective properties. The majority of these studies are seeking effective and nontoxic agents for use in radiation therapy for cancer, as synthetic compounds for such purposes are toxic at their optimal concentrations. We can extrapolate that if various plant species have radioprotective effects for such purposes that they would probably be beneficial for protecting ourselves from radionuclides as well.

There is a crucial distinction to be made between the terms "radioprotective," which is based on protecting the body from the damaging effects of ionizing radiation, both internally and externally, and "detoxification," which assumes that elements such as plutonium and cesium can be "decorporated," or flushed out of the system. If such detoxification can occur, it would be done through chelation.

Every radioactive element not only has a specific affinity for certain organs and tissues, but also has different biochemical routes and rates of excretion. There is a large amount of academic research available about synthetic chelating agents for various metals, including some of the radionuclides, but the status of the science appears the same as synthetic radioprotective agents: poorly understood, highly toxic, and relatively inefficient.

On the other hand, there are numerous articles circulating in the field of natural health about "detoxification" of radiation. The majority of these appear to have some good suggestions, such as eating healthy foods high in antioxidants, but they also propose therapies that are based on a rather simplistic understanding of the complexities of the subject; for example, one of the widely circulated regimens for treatment of radiation involves baking soda baths and internal ingestion of clay.

Surprisingly, other than a very short list of potential candidates, research substantiating the effectiveness and mechanisms of natural chelators appears to be lacking. In researching the effectiveness of baking soda for chelation as baths or taken orally, for example, I found no studies that offer any evidence that it works in the tissues at a biochemical level or that excretion rates can be measured. I found instead that sodium bicarbonate has indeed been used as a chelating agent for uranium toxicity of the kidneys, but it must be given intravenously and has poor results. (6) A few studies have been done with encouraging results using seaweeds and alginate from seaweeds, pectins and a handful of other items, which will be discussed at the end of this section; overall, however, the field of natural chelation appears to be poorly developed.

Rather than repeat natural health information about "detoxification" that may be generally beneficial but is lacking in medical substantiation, I have chosen the more tedious route of analyzing the academic studies of the in vivo and in vitro effects of gamma radiation on mice, most of which examine the survival rates and the various types of radioprotection that plants may give against cellular damage. While many students, including myself, find such studies odious, what emerges are valuable pieces of information about the various modes of biochemical and physiological actions through which herbs give their protective effects; by understanding these modes of action we can further develop a pharmacopeia to include other botanical species that have those actions, even if they have not been studied specifically for this purpose.

Radioprotective Herbs and Foods

This is a short list of some of the representative herbs and foods that have confirmed radioprotective powers, with notes on their likely mechanisms of action. Some of these also have known chelating effects.

Ginseng

Several studies have been done on ginsengs. Panax quinquefolius, American ginseng, was found to have post irradiation protective effects on human lymphocytes. Its mechanism of action appears to be scavenging of free radicals and enhancement of intracellular antioxidant capacity. (7)

Panax ginseng has been found to "reduce cell damage caused by gamma-rays, especially damage to DNA molecules, and play a role in the repair or regeneration process of damaged cells." (8)

The activity levels of various ginsenosides have been studied for their abilities to inhibit cell death and stimulate cell formation after irradiation. (9)

The ginsenoside panaxadiol is thought to have the major radioprotective effect. (10)

Decoction of whole Panax ginseng root has been found to give better radioprotective effects against DNA damage than individual ginsenosides. Its mechanisms of action can be attributed to what is traditionally known about its immunomodulatory, antimutagenic and adaptogenic activities. (11)

Rhodiola

The high altitude Himalayan plant Rhodiola imbricate was found to give in vitro and in vivo radioprotection through a synergisitic effect of superoxide ion scavenging, metal chelation, antioxidant, anti-lipid peroxidation and anti-hemolytic activities. (12)

Cordyceps

Cordyceps is a medicinal fungus used for increasing endurance and immunity. Water extract was found to have radioprotective effects against gamma radiation on bone marrow and the intestines, increased survival rates, and caused rapid recovery of white blood cell levels. One of its proposed mechanisms is reduction of free radicals within cells. (13)

Cordyceps was also found to create a dose dependent increase in leucocyte levels, and to promote return to normal baseline levels after gamma irradiation. It doubled lymphocyte levels and significantly increased survival rates after lethal doses of radiation. (14)

Centella asiatica

Gotu kola has a well established reputation as a rejuvenative herb in Ayurveda. It has been found to reduce weight loss and increase survival time of irradiated mice. (15)

Gotu kola has been found to significantly reduce damage to DNA, reduce lipid peroxidation, prevent radiation induced decline of antioxidant enzyme levels, and reduce mortality after whole body radiation. (16)

Centella was found to protect hepatocytes from radiation damage. (17)

Chyavanprash

Chyavanprash is an Ayurvedic rejuvenative herbal preparation based on Emblica officinalis. Its use delayed symptoms of radiation sickness, gave significant protection to the GI tract and bones, and increased survival rates at low doses. (18)

Triphala

Triphala is a famous Ayurvedic formula used as a mild bowel tonic and rejuvenative, among many others uses. It was found to have a dose dependent radio-protective effect against radiation sickness and mortality. (19)

Triphala provided protection against both GI and hemopoietic mortality, and increased tolerance to higher doses of gamma radiation. Its mechanism of action was found to be free radical scavenging. (20)

Emblica officinalis

Amla is a major rejuvenative nutritive herb in Ayurveda, and one of the highest sources of vitamin C. Administered before exposure to gamma radiation, it was found to be protective of peripheral blood chemistry. It produced a significant increase of white and red blood cells, hemoglobin and hematocrit values, and reduced radiation sickness. Reduced glutathione levels were increased and lipid peroxidation levels decreased. (21)

Amla increased survival time, reduced weight loss and mortality of irradiated mice. (22)

Hippophae rhamnoides

Numerous studies have been done on the radioprotective effects of sea buckthorn. A tincture of the whole berries was found to protect DNA strands from gamma radiation, attributed primarily to direct modulation of chromatin compaction and organization. (23) (24)

Sea buckthorn extract was found to have antioxidant radioprotective effects on DNA at higher doses, but at lower doses it acted in the opposite way, damaging DNA as a prooxidant. (25)

Another study found that sea buckthorn extract protected DNA of the mitochondria and genomes from radiation induced damage, which was attributed to the free radical scavenging of its polyphenols and flavonoids. (26)

Sea buckthorn extract gave an 82% survival rate after whole body gamma radiation, compared to no survival in the control group. The results were attributed to free radical scavenging, acceleration of stem cell proliferation and immunostimulation. (27)

Sea buckthorn extract was found to have immunostimulant actions by maintaining macrophage and splenocyte counts. (28)

Treatment with sea buckthorn extract was found to protect spermatogenesis by enhancing spermatogonial proliferation, enhancing stem cell survival and reducing sperm abnormalities; its actions were attributed to free radical scavenging and the presence of polyphenolic flavonoids. (29)

The radioprotective actions of sea buckthorn were attributed to its flavonoid content such as quercetin. (30)

Aloe Vera

Aloe very leaf extract administered to mice was found to have damage-resistant properties against whole body gamma radiation-induced biochemical alterations. Its radioprotective actions are attributed to increasing superoxide dismutase in the skin and glutathione in the liver and blood, and decreasing lipid peroxidation in the liver and blood. (31)

Boerhaavia diffusa

Boerhaavia is an important Ayurvedic herb, used primarily as a diuretic for conditions of stagnant fluids and for pain relief. The whole plant extract has been found to have protective effects against gamma radiation induced damage in mice, primarily through preventing decrease of white blood cells, lowering levels of lipid peroxidation and protecting bone marrow DNA. Elevated levels of alkaline phosphatase, frequently cited as a response to irradiation as well as being found in some cancers, were reduced. (32)

Adhatoda vasica

Adhatoda vasica is an important herb used in Ayurveda, primarily for treating respiratory infections and expectorating phlegm. The leaf extract was found to have a modulatory influence against radiation induced hematological alterations in mice. 100% of the untreated control group died within twenty-five days after irradiation, while there was an 81% survival rate in the treated group. The treated group had significantly higher levels of reduced glutathione and lower levels of lipid peroxidation. (33)

In another study it was found that pretreatment of irradiated mice with Adhatoda extract increased survival rates, significantly prevented radiation-induced chromosomal damage in bone marrow cells, and had significant radioprotective effects on testis tissue architecture and various cell populations including spermatogonia (undifferentiated sperm cells), spermatids and Leydig cells. The usual findings about elevated levels of reduced glutathione and lowered levels of lipid peroxidation were also noted. (34)

Curcumin

Curcumin is a major phytochemical compound found in turmeric. It has been found to reduce injury and fibrosis to the lungs caused by radiation. Its therapeutic action is attributed to prevention or modulation of inflammation and oxidative stress. (35)

Piper longum

Long pepper is an important herb used in Ayurveda, primarily as a warming digestive stimulant and respiratory expectorant. The tincture of Piper longum fruit had radioprotective effects on irradiated mice. Its primary mechanism of actions was maintaining white blood cell levels, enhancing bone marrow cells and increasing the production of reduced glutathione, the major endogenous antioxidant produced by the cells, and reducing elevated levels of lipid peroxidation. (36)

Acorus calamus

Calamus root is an important herb used in Ayurveda, specifically as an aromatic cerebral stimulant tonic. Acorus extract was found to decrease the number of breaks in DNA strands and increase survival rates of irradiated mice. Its mechanism of action was increasing the activities of major enzymes of the antioxidant defense system. (37)

Mentha piperita

Peppermint leaf extract was found to have modulatory and protective effects on the histology, lipid peroxidation, and phosphatase levels in testis. The untreated control group had decrease of testis weight, severe testicular atrophy and degeneration of germ cells; in contrast, the treated group had increase of testis weight, normal testicular morphology and germ cells. The results were attributed to the high amounts of phenolic and flavonoid compounds found in peppermint, and their antioxidant and radical scavenging activity. (38) (39)

Peppermint was found to have a radioprotective effect against chromosomal damage in bone marrow from gamma radiation. (40)

Mentha arvensis

Mint extract was found to have a dose dependent radioprotective effect against gamma radiation exposure. It reduced the severity of radiation sickness and mortality. (41)

Rosemarinus officinalis

Rosemary was found to have the usual radioprotective effects of lessening radiation sickness and increasing survival rates, with the typical findings of increasing glutathione and reducing lipid peroxidation levels. (42)

Zingiber officinale

Extracts of ginger have been found to have protective effects against gamma radiation inducted sickness and mortality, that have been attributed to its free radical scavenging, antioxidant, anti-inflammatory and anti-mutagenic effects. Its actions were specifically protective of the GI tract and bone marrow. It has also been found to selectively protect normal tissues against the tumoricidal effects of radiation treatments. (43) (44) (45)

Ocinum sanctum

A polysaccharide isolated from Ocinum sanctum was found to prevent oxidative damage from gamma radiation; it had free radical scavenging effects, and could prevent splenocyte cell deaths. (46)

Holy basil extract was found to give in vivo protection against chromosome damage from radiation in mice, and faster recovery than untreated animals; free radical scavenging was the proposed mechanism of action. (47)

Two flavonoids from leaves of Ocinum sanctum were found to significantly reduce chromosomal aberrations at low doses and with no toxicity. (48)

Other species of basils have also been found to have radioprotective effects (Ocimum gratissimum, Ocimum basilicum, Ocimum canum, and Ocimum kilimandscharicum). The extracts had modulatory effects against gamma radiation induced chromosomal damage, and increased the levels of reduced glutathione. (49)

Seaweed

Different species of seaweeds have been analyzed for their radioprotective properties. Extracts of red seaweed (Callophyllis japonica) increased survival rates after gamma radiation exposure up to 80%, possibly due to protection of hematopoietic and intestinal stem cells. (50)

A component of brown seaweed (Ecklonia cava) significantly reduced mortality of lethally irradiated mice; its mechanisms were determined to be improved hematopoietic recovery, repair of damaged DNA, and enhancement of immune cells. (51)

Chlorella

Chlorella increased the number of hemopoietic stem cells in bone marrow and spleen, increasing survival rates of irradiated mice. (52)

Spirulina

Spirulina produced radioprotective effect through differenct mechanism in mice and dogs. It increased the level of white and nucleated cells and DNA in bone marrow in mice; in dogs it increased the levels of red and white cells, hemoglobins and nucleated cells in bone marrow. (53)

Miso

Miso was found to have radioprotective effects, with the greatest effects produced by miso that had fermented the longest. (54)

Placenta Extract

Placenta has been used traditionally in Chinese medicine for nutritive and strengthening purposes; it has probably been used throughout history in other cultures as well. Deer and goat placenta are found in modern Chinese herbal products with tonifying and strengthening powers for rebuilding core vitality in cases of severe nutritional depletion.

Research conducted at the Atomic Bomb Disease Institute at Nagasaki University has found that placenta extract "significantly attenuated the acute radiation injury to bone marrow-derived stem/progenitor cells, and this protection is likely to be related to the anti-inflammatory activity of the placental extract." (55)

Chelating Agents

Below is a short list of natural chelating agents that have benefits substantiated by in vivo research. While I am very familiar and well versed with the uses of the herbs listed above, these are substances that I know little about and have no clinical experience with; this information is offered for further research purposes and not specific therapeutic applications.

Sodium Alginate

A flavorless polysaccharide gum extracted from various types of seaweeds, alginate has been found to be an effective chelator that prevents assimilation of radionuclides in the GI tract.

Sodium alginate can be prepared from different species of algae such as Sargassum and different species of seaweeds such as Laminaria. Sodium alginate prepared from Sargassum siliquastrum was found to be highly effective for reducing absorption of radioactive strontium with virtually no toxicity, disruption of digestive function, or disturbance of mineral metabolism. It has been suggested that alginate can be added to the diet or used as a syrup for immediate chelation. (56)

The addition of alginate reduced the absorption of radioactive strontium in milk by a factor of nine. (57)

Low doses of sodium alginate were found to significantly reduce the uptake of radioactive strontium into bones. (58)

Apple Pectin

A number of studies have found that apple pectin added to the diet has a chelating effect on cesium. (59)

Apple pectin was given to children exposed to radioactive fallout from Chernobyl. It was found that it significantly reduced the levels of cesium 137, even in a radiologically clean environment with a radiologically clean diet, indicating that it worked to chelate the cesium from the tissues and not simply prevent its absorption in the GI tract. (60)

In a contradictory study comparing the effectiveness of apple pectin with Prussian blue for chelation of cesium 137 in rats, it was found that the pectin had no significant effects, but the Prussian blue produced a five-fold increase of fecal excretion of the cesium. (61)

Prussian Blue

Prussian blue is an iron-based pigment that is regarded as a relatively non-toxic chelating agent for removing cesium 137. When formulated correctly, it is considered by the FDA to be a safe and effective therapy for certain cases of poisoning; the International Atomic Energy Agency states that up to ten grams a day can be consumed safely. It is sold commercially in Russia in soluble capsules for chelating cesium. Its mechanism appears to be sequestering of heavy metals and removing them from the GI tract and indirectly from hepatic circulation. (62)

Prussian blue was used for decontamination of cesium 137 in thirty-nine people exposed during an incident where radioactive material was stolen from a facility in Brazil. It caused dose reductions averaging 71 percent. (63)

In a second study after that incident it was found that Prussian blue appeared to reduce the half-life of cesium by 32 percent, and that the optimum dosage was dependent on individual weight. (64)

Prussian blue is described as "a crystal lattice that exchanges potassium for cesium at the surface of the crystal." Its mechanism is to bind cesium in the gut before it can be reabsorbed. Other studies have found that it can reduce the half-life of cesium by 43 percent and reduce overall body burden of that element. (65)

Conclusion

In reading these studies, we should remember that many animals suffered and died in order for this information to be gathered. In a way, they are a metaphor for the larger experiment that is being done on humanity by the nuclear industry and its close relationship with the military. As practitioners, we should regard the use of herbs for radioprotective purposes as a superficial, symptomatic and temporary treatment of a much deeper disease, a disease that has political, environmental and spiritual dimensions.

References

(1) http://en.wikipedia.org/wiki/List_of_military_nuclear_accidents
(2) http://en.wikipedia.org/wiki/List_of_nuclear_reactors
(3) http://en.wikipedia.org/wiki/Nuclear_and_radiation_accidents
(4) http://en.wikipedia.org/wiki/List_of_nuclear_tests
(5) Fukushima Accident: Radioactive Releases and Potential Dose Consequences
Peter F. Caracappa, Ph.D., CHP; Rensselaer Polytechnic Institute
ANS Annual Meeting Special Session: The Accident at Fukushima Daiichi— Preliminary Investigations
June 28, 2011
(6) Radiat Prot Dosimetry. 2007;127(1-4):477-9. Epub 2007 Jul 12.
Inositol hexaphosphate: a potential chelating agent for uranium.
Cebrian D, Tapia A, Real A, Morcillo MA.
Radiobiology Laboratory, Radiation Dosimetry Unit, Department of Environment, CIEMAT, Avda Complutense 22, 28040 Madrid, Spain.
(7) J Altern Complement Med. 2010 May;16(5):561-7. doi: 10.1089/acm.2009.0590.

Radioprotective effect of American ginseng on human lymphocytes at 90 minutes postirradiation: a study of 40 cases.

Lee TK, O'Brien KF, Wang W, Johnke RM, Sheng C, Benhabib SM, Wang T, Allison RR.

Department of Radiation Oncology, Leo W. Jenkins Cancer Center, Brody School of Medicine at East Carolina University, Greenville, NC, USA.

(8) In Vivo. 1993 Sep-Oct;7(5):467-70.

In vivo radioprotective activity of Panax ginseng and diethyldithiocarbamate.

Kim SH, Cho CK, Yoo SY, Koh KH, Yun HG, Kim TH.

Laboratory of Radiation Medicine, Korea Cancer Center Hospital, Seoul.

(9) Phytother Res. 2006 May;20(5):392-5.

In Vivo radioprotective effect of Panax ginseng C.A. Meyer and identification of active ginsenosides.

Lee HJ, Kim SR, Kim JC, Kang CM, Lee YS, Jo SK, Kim TH, Jang JS, Nah SY, Kim SH.

College of Veterinary Medicine, Chonnam National University, Gwangju, South Korea.

(10) In Vivo. 2003 Jan-Feb;17(1):77-81.

Modification of radiation response in mice by ginsenosides, active components of Panax ginseng.

Kim SR, Jo SK, Kim SH.

Department of Anatomy, College of Veterinary Medicine, Chonnam National University, 300 Yongbong-dong, Puk-ku, Kwangju 500-757, South Korea.

(11) Radioprotective potential of ginseng.

Lee TK, Johnke RM, Allison RR, O'Brien KF, Dobbs LJ Jr.

Department of Radiation Oncology, Leo W. Jenkins Cancer Center, Brody School of Medicine at East Carolina University, Greenville, NC 27858, USA.

(12) Mol Cell Biochem. 2005 May;273(1-2):209-23.

Evaluation of radioprotective activities Rhodiola imbricata Edgew--a high altitude plant.

Arora R, Chawla R, Sagar R, Prasad J, Singh S, Kumar R, Sharma A, Singh S, Sharma RK.

Division of Radiopharmaceuticals and Radiation Biology, Institute of Nuclear Medicine and Allied Sciences, Delhi, India

(13) Radiat Res. 2006 Dec;166(6):900-7.

Protection against radiation-induced bone marrow and intestinal injuries by Cordyceps sinensis, a Chinese herbal medicine.

Liu WC, Wang SC, Tsai ML, Chen MC, Wang YC, Hong JH, McBride

WH, Chiang CS.

Department of Biomedical Engineering and Environmental Sciences, National Tsing Hua University, Hsinchu 30013, Taiwan.

(14) Int J Radiat Biol. 2008 Feb;84(2):139-49. doi: 10.1080/09553000701797070.

Radiation mitigation effect of cultured mushroom fungus Hirsutella Sinensis (CorImmune) isolated from a Chinese/Tibetan herbal preparation -Cordyceps Sinensis.

Xun C, Shen N, Li B, Zhang Y, Wang F, Yang Y, Shi X, Schafermyer K, Brown SA, Thompson JS.

Division of Hematology/Oncology, Department of Medicine, Veterans Affairs Medical Center and University of Kentucky Medical Center, Lexington, Kentucky, USA.

(15) Phytother Res. 2002 Dec;16(8):785-6.

Radioprotection of Swiss albino mouse by Centella asiatica extract.

Sharma J, Sharma R.

Department of Zoology, University of Rajasthan, Jaipur 302004, India.

(16) J Pharm Pharmacol. 2009 Jul;61(7):941-7. doi: 10.1211/jpp/61.07.0014.

Protection of DNA and membranes from gamma-radiation induced damages by Centella asiatica.

Joy J, Nair CK.

Amala Cancer Research Centre, Kerala, India.

(17) Phytother Res. 2005 Jul;19(7):605-11.

Modification of gamma ray induced changes in the mouse hepatocytes by Centella asiatica extract: in vivo studies.

Sharma R, Sharma J.

Department of Zoology, University of Rajasthan, Jaipur 302004, India.

(18) Phytother Res. 2004 Jan;18(1):14-8.

The evaluation of the radioprotective effect of chyavanaprasha (an ayurvedic rasayana drug) in mice exposed to lethal dose of gamma-radiation: a preliminary study.

Jagetia GC, Baliga MS.

Department of Radiobiology, Kasturba Medical College, Manipal, India.

(19) Phytomedicine. 2002 Mar;9(2):99-108.

The evaluation of the radioprotective effect of Triphala (an ayurvedic rejuvenating drug) in the mice exposed to gamma-radiation.

Jagetia GC, Baliga MS, Malagi KJ, Sethukumar Kamath M.

Department of Radiobiology, Kasturba Medical College, Manipal, India.

(20) J Altern Complement Med. 2004 Dec;10(6):971-8.

Triphala, an ayurvedic rasayana drug, protects mice against radiation-induced lethality by free-radical scavenging.

Jagetia GC, Malagi KJ, Baliga MS, Venkatesh P, Veruva RR.

Department of Radiobiology, Kasturba Medical College, Manipal-576 104, Karnataka, India.

(21) J Environ Pathol Toxicol Oncol. 2006;25(4):643-54.

Emblica officinalis (Linn.) fruit extract provides protection against radiation-induced hematological and biochemical alterations in mice.

Singh I, Soyal D, Goyal PK.

Radiation and Cancer Biology Laboratory, Department of Zoology, University of Rajasthan, Jaipur, India.

(22) Phytother Res. 2005 May;19(5):444-6.

Radioprotection of Swiss albino mice by Emblica officinalis.

Singh I, Sharma A, Nunia V, Goyal PK.

Radiation and Cancer Biology Laboratory, Department of Zoology, University of Rajasthan, Jaipur 302 004, India.

(23) Mol Cell Biochem. 2002 Sep;238(1-2):1-9.

Modulation of chromatin organization by RH-3, a preparation of Hippophae rhamnoides, a possible role in radioprotection.

Kumar IP, Namita S, Goel HC.

Department of Radiation Biology, Institute of Nuclear Medicine and Allied Sciences, INMAS, Delhi, India.

(24) Mol Cell Biochem. 2003 Mar;245(1-2):57-67.

Induction of DNA-protein cross-links by Hippophae rhamnoides: implications in radioprotection and cytotoxicity.

Goel HC, Kumar IP, Samanta N, Rana SV.

Department of Radiation Biology, Institute of Nuclear Medicine and Allied Sciences, Brig S.K. Majumdar Marg, Delhi, India.

(25) J Environ Pathol Toxicol Oncol. 2004;23(2):123-37.

Induction of apoptosis in thymocytes by Hippophae rhamnoides: implications in radioprotection.

Goel HC, Indraghanti P, Samanta N, Ranaz SV.

Department of Radiation Biology, Institute of Nuclear Medicine and Allied Sciences, Delhi, India.

(26) Environ Mol Mutagen. 2006 Dec;47(9):647-56.

Protection from radiation-induced mitochondrial and genomic DNA damage by an extract of Hippophae rhamnoides.

Shukla SK, Chaudhary P, Kumar IP, Samanta N, Afrin F, Gupta ML, Sharma UK, Sinha AK, Sharma YK, Sharma RK.

Division of Radioimaging, Bioinformatics, and Radiation Biology, Institute of Nuclear Medicine and Allied Sciences, Delhi, India.

(27) Phytomedicine. 2002 Jan;9(1):15-25.

Radioprotection by a herbal preparation of Hippophae rhamnoides, RH-3, against whole body lethal irradiation in mice.

Goel HC, Prasad J, Singh S, Sagar RK, Kumar IP, Sinha AK.

Department of Radiation Biology, Institute of Nuclear medicine and Allied Sciences, Delhi, India.

(28) J Pharm Pharmacol. 2005 Aug;57(8):1065-72.

Modification of gamma radiation induced response of peritoneal macrophages and splenocytes by Hippophae rhamnoides (RH-3) in mice.

Prakash H, Bala M, Ali A, Goel HC.

Department of Radiation Biology, Institute of Nuclear Medicine and Allied Sciences, Brig S.K. Mazumdar Marg, Delhi-110054, India.

(29) Andrologia. 2006 Dec;38(6):199-207.

Protection of spermatogenesis in mice against gamma ray induced damage by Hippophae rhamnoides.

Goel HC, Samanta N, Kannan K, Kumar IP, Bala M.

Department of Microbiology, Chaudhary Charan Singh University, Meerut, UP, India.

(30) J Med Food. 2007 Mar;10(1):101-9.

Radioprotective and antioxidant activity of fractionated extracts of berries of Hippophae rhamnoides.

Chawla R, Arora R, Singh S, Sagar RK, Sharma RK, Kumar R, Sharma A, Gupta ML, Singh S, Prasad J, Khan HA, Swaroop A, Sinha AK, Gupta AK, Tripathi RP, Ahuja PS.

Institute of Nuclear Medicine and Allied Sciences, Defence Research and Development Organization, Jamia Hamdard, Hamdard Nagar, Delhi, India.

(31) J Environ Pathol Toxicol Oncol. 2009;28(1):53-61.

Radioprotective effects of Aloe vera leaf extract on Swiss albino mice against whole-body gamma irradiation.

Goyal PK, Gehlot P.

Department of Zoology, University of Rajasthan, Jaipur - 302 004, India.

(32) Integr Cancer Ther. 2007 Dec;6(4):381-8.

Studies on the protective effects of Boerhaavia diffusa L. against gamma radiation induced damage in mice.

Manu KA, Leyon PV, Kuttan G.
Amala Cancer Research Centre, Amala Nagar, Kerala State, India.
(33) Phytomedicine. 2005 Apr;12(4):285-93.
Modulatory influence of Adhatoda vasica Nees leaf extract against gamma irradiation in Swiss albino mice.
Kumar A, Ram J, Samarth RM, Kumar M.
Radiation and Cancer Biology Laboratory, Department of Zoology, University of Rajasthan, Jaipur, India.
(34) Evid Based Complement Alternat Med. 2007 Sep;4(3):343-50.
Protective effect of Adhatoda vascia Nees against radiation-induced damage at cellular, biochemical and chromosomal levels in Swiss albino mice.
Kumar M, Samarth R, Kumar M, Selvan SR, Saharan B, Kumar A.
Laboratory of Radiation and Cancer Biology, Department of Zoology, University of Rajasthan Jaipur 302004, India.
(35) Protection from acute and chronic lung diseases by curcumin
Author Venkatesan N., Punithavathi D., Babu M.
Journal Advances in Experimental Medicine and Biology
Issue ID 595; Page 379-405; Date 2007
(36) Protective effect of Piper longum fruit ethanolic extract on radiation induced damages in mice: a preliminary study.
Sunila ES, Kuttan G.
Amala Cancer Research Centre, Trissur, India.
(37) Exp Toxicol Pathol. 2012 Jan;64(1-2):57-64. doi: 10.1016/j.etp.2010.06.006. Epub 2010 Jul 5.
Protection from lethal and sub-lethal whole body exposures of mice to γ-radiation by Acorus calamus L.: studies on tissue antioxidant status and cellular DNA damage.
Sandeep D, Nair CK.
Amala Cancer Research Centre, Amala nagar, Trichur 680555, Kerala, India.
(38) Basic Clin Pharmacol Toxicol. 2009 Apr;104(4):329-34. doi: 10.1111/j.1742-7843.2009.00384.x.
Protection against radiation-induced testicular damage in Swiss albino mice by Mentha piperita (Linn.).
Samarth RM, Samarth M.
Radiation and Cancer Biology Laboratory, Department of Zoology, University of Rajasthan, Jaipur 302055, India.
(39) J Cancer Res Ther. 2010 Jul-Sep;6(3):255-62. doi: 10.4103/0973-1482.73336.

Radioprotective potential of mint: a brief review.

Baliga MS, Rao S.

Research and Development, Father Muller Medical College, Father Muller Hospital Road, Kankanady, Mangalore, India. research@gmail.com

(40) Indian J Exp Biol. 2003 Mar;41(3):229-37.

Mentha piperita (Linn.) leaf extract provides protection against radiation induced chromosomal damage in bone marrow of mice.

Samarth RM, Kumar A.

Radiation & Cancer Biology Laboratory, Department of Zoology, University of Rajasthan, Jaipur 302004, India.

(41) Strahlenther Onkol. 2002 Feb;178(2):91-8.

Influence of the leaf extract of Mentha arvensis Linn. (mint) on the survival of mice exposed to different doses of gamma radiation.

Jagetia GC, Baliga MS.

Department of Radiobiology, Kasturba Medical College, Manipal, India.

(42) J Environ Pathol Toxicol Oncol. 2006;25(4):633-42.

Radioprotective potential of Rosemarinus officinalis against lethal effects of gamma radiation : a preliminary study.

Jindal A, Soyal D, Sancheti G, Goyal PK.

Radiation and Cancer Biology Laboratory, Department of Zoology, University of Rajasthan, Jaipur - 302 004, India.

(43) Food Funct. 2012 Jul;3(7):714-23. doi: 10.1039/c2fo10225k. Epub 2012 May 18.

Radioprotective effects of Zingiber officinale Roscoe (ginger): past, present and future.

Baliga MS, Haniadka R, Pereira MM, Thilakchand KR, Rao S, Arora R.

Research and Development, Father Muller Medical College, Father Muller Hospital Road, Kankanady, Mangalore, Karnataka, India 575002.

(44) Radiat Res. 2003 Nov;160(5):584-92.

Influence of ginger rhizome (Zingiber officinale Rosc) on survival, glutathione and lipid peroxidation in mice after whole-body exposure to gamma radiation.

Jagetia GC, Baliga MS, Venkatesh P, Ulloor JN.

Department of Radiobiology, Kasturba Medical College, Manipal 576 119, India.

(45) Cancer Biother Radiopharm. 2004 Aug;19(4):422-35.

Ginger (Zingiber officinale Rosc.), a dietary supplement, protects mice against radiation-induced lethality: mechanism of action.

Jagetia G, Baliga M, Venkatesh P.
Department of Radiobiology, Kasturba Medical College, Manipal, India.
(46) Redox Rep. 2005;10(5):257-64.
Antioxidant and radioprotective properties of an Ocimum sanctum polysaccharide.
Subramanian M, Chintalwar GJ, Chattopadhyay S.
Bio-Organic Division, Bhabha Atomic Research Centre, Mumbai, India.
(47) Mutat Res. 1997 Feb 3;373(2):271-6.
Protection against radiation-induced chromosome damage in mouse bone marrow by Ocimum sanctum.
Ganasoundari A, Devi PU, Rao MN.
Department of Radiobiology, Dr. T.M.A. Pai Research Centre, Kasturba Medical College, Manipal, India.
(48) Br J Radiol. 1998 Jul;71(847):782-4.
A comparative study of radioprotection by Ocimum flavonoids and synthetic aminothiol protectors in the mouse.
Devi PU, Bisht KS, Vinitha M.
Department of Radiobiology, Kasturba Medical College, Manipal, India.
(49) Pharm Biol. 2011 Apr;49(4):428-36. doi:
10.3109/13880209.2010.521513.
Antimelanoma and radioprotective activity of alcoholic aqueous extract of different species of Ocimum in C(57)BL mice.
Monga J, Sharma M, Tailor N, Ganesh N.
Research Department, Jawaharlal Nehru Cancer Hospital and Research Center, Idgah Hills, Bhopal, Madhya Pradesh, India.
(50) J Vet Sci. 2008 Sep;9(3):281-4.
The radioprotective effects of the hexane and ethyl acetate extracts of Callophyllis japonica in mice that undergo whole body irradiation.
Kim J, Moon C, Kim H, Jeong J, Lee J, Kim J, Hyun JW, Park JW, Moon MY, Lee NH, Kim SH, Jee Y, Shin T.
College of Veterinary Medicine, and the Research Institute for Subtropical Agriculture and Biotechnology, Cheju National University, Jeju 690-756, Korea.
(51) Radioprotective properties of eckol against ionizing radiation in mice
Edited by Vladimir Skulachev; Eunjin Park, Gin-nae Ahn, Nam Ho Lee, Jeong Mi Kim, Jin Seok Yun, Jin Won Hyun, You-Jin Jeon, Myung Bok Wie, Young Jae Lee, Jae Woo Park, Youngheun Jee
(52) Strahlenther Onkol. 1989 Nov;165(11):813-6.

The radioprotective effects of aqueous extract from chlorococcal freshwater algae (Chlorella kessleri) in mice and rats.

Rotkovská D, Vacek A, Bartoníčková A.

Institute of Biophysics, Czechoslovak Academy of Sciences, Brno.

(53) Acta Pharmacol Sin. 2001 Dec;22(12):1121-4.

Chemo- and radio-protective effects of polysaccharide of Spirulina platensis on hemopoietic system of mice and dogs.

Zhang HQ, Lin AP, Sun Y, Deng YM.

The Medical and Pharmaceutical Academe of Yangzhou University, Yangzhou 225001, China.

(54) Hiroshima J Med Sci. 2001 Dec;50(4):83-6.

Radioprotective effects of miso (fermented soy bean paste) against radiation in B6C3F1 mice: increased small intestinal crypt survival, crypt lengths and prolongation of average time to death.

Ohara M, Lu H, Shiraki K, Ishimura Y, Uesaka T, Katoh O, Watanabe H.

Department of Environment and Mutation, Research Institute for Radiation Biology and Medicine, Hiroshima University, Japan.

(55) J Radiat Res. 2012 Nov 14. [Epub ahead of print]

Placental extract protects bone marrow-derived stem/progenitor cells against radiation injury through anti-inflammatory activity.

Kawakatsu M, Urata Y, Goto S, Ono Y, Li TS.

Department of Stem Cell Biology, Atomic Bomb Disease Institute, Nagasaki University Graduate School of Biomedical Science, 1-12-4 Sakamoto, Nagasaki 852-8523, Japan.

(56) Biomed Environ Sci. 1991 Sep;4(3):273-82.

Suppression of radioactive strontium absorption by sodium alginate in animals and human subjects.

Gong YF, Huang ZJ, Qiang MY, Lan FX, Bai GA, Mao YX, Ma XP, Zhang FG.

Institute of Radiation Medicine, Beijing, China.

(57) Health Phys. 2004 Feb;86(2):193-6. Strontium biokinetics in humans: influence of alginate on the uptake of ingested strontium.

Höllriegl V, Röhmuss M, Oeh U, Roth P. GSF-National Research Centre for Environment and Health, Institute of Radiation Protection, Ingolstadter Landstrasse 1, D-85764, Neuherberg, Germany.

(58) Can Med Assoc J. 1965 Aug 28;93:404-7.

Studies of inhibition of intestinal absorption of Radioactive Strontium. IV. estimation of the suppressant effect of sodium alginate.

Skoryna SC, Paul TM, Waldron-Edward D.
(59) Swiss Med Wkly. 2004 Dec 18;134(49-50):725-9.
Relationship between caesium (137Cs) load, cardiovascular symptoms, and source of food in 'Chernobyl' children -- preliminary observations after intake of oral apple pectin.
Bandazhevskaya GS, Nesterenko VB, Babenko VI, Yerkovich TV, Bandazhevsky YI.
Institute of Radiation Safety Belrad, Minsk, Republic of Belarus.
(60) Swiss Med Wkly. 2004 Jan 10;134(1-2):24-7.
Reducing the 137Cs-load in the organism of "Chernobyl" children with apple-pectin.
Nesterenko VB, Nesterenko AV, Babenko VI, Yerkovich TV, Babenko IV.
Belrad Institute of Radiation Safety, Charity House, 11 Staroborisovsky Trakt, 220114 Minsk, Republic of Belarus.
(61) Biochimie. 2006 Nov;88(11):1837-41. Epub 2006 Sep 28.
Comparison of Prussian blue and apple-pectin efficacy on 137Cs decorporation in rats.
Le Gall B, Taran F, Renault D, Wilk JC, Ansoborlo E.
CEA/DSV/DRR/SRCA/LRT, Bruyères-le-Châtel, France.
(62) http://en.wikipedia.org/wiki/Prussian_blue
(63) Health Phys. 1994 Mar;66(3):245-52.
137Cs internal contamination involving a Brazilian accident, and the efficacy of Prussian Blue treatment.
Melo DR, Lipsztein JL, de Oliveira CA, Bertelli L.
Instituto de Radioproteção e Dosimetria/CNEN, Barra da Tijuca-Rio de Janeiro/RJ, Brasil.
(64) Health Phys. 1991 Jan;60(1):57-61.
Studies of Cs retention in the human body related to body parameters and Prussian blue administration.
Lipsztein JL, Bertelli L, Oliveira CA, Dantas BM.
Instituto de Radioproteção e Dosimetria/CNEN, Rio de Janeiro, Brazil.
(65) Pharmacotherapy. 2001 Nov;21(11):1364-7.
Prussian blue for treatment of radiocesium poisoning.
Thompson DF, Church CO.
Department Pharmacy Practice, Southwestern Oklahoma State University, Weatherford, USA.

IV

Stimulants
The Upsides and Downsides

Introduction

When I first started writing this article I had a simple idea in mind: compare some of the benefits and disadvantages of common herbal stimulants such as yerba mate, tea, coffee and a few others. As my research progressed, I began to feel that I have been leading a sheltered life, and that without noticing had become a naïve herbal elder who knew nothing about what was really going on in modern culture.

A brave new world of stimulation was all around me, a world I was somehow out of touch with. I knew from clinical experience that people get addicted to caffeine and that aspartame in diet sodas gives a nasty and prolonged withdrawal. But here was a vast new selection of legal stimulants I had missed out on, available at every corner market: Red Bull, Pimp Juice, Cocaine, Rockstar, Spike Shooter, Redline, Monster Assault. My customary preferences for adrenal titillation began to look rather innocent, even healthy.

I have treated many cases of stimulant addiction, from coke snorters to crack smokers to meth shooters, but even that was outdated. Here was a veritable cornucopia of new amphetamine and ecstasy-like psychostimulants just waiting to be sampled, knowingly or unknowingly, by anyone going to a typical college party.

I have some experience and expertise with the rejuvenative, tonifying and adaptogenic botanicals of Ayurvedic and Chinese medicine. But here was an aspect of society that I knew practically nothing about: herbal stimulants combined with a myriad other compounds and amino acids of every flavor, for enhancement of everything we could possibly feel inadequate about. Performance enhancers for working out at the gym, thermogenic enhancers for losing real or imaginary weight, brain enhancers for those wanting more mental focus and clarity, sexual enhancers for those of flagging libido, all with chat groups and online forums to discuss dosages and side effects and personal discoveries and the occasional hospitalization incident.

My brief and somewhat academic contact with popular culture was an eye opening experience, not just from seeing the range of new stimulants available to everyone since I last checked, but their incredible toxicity, the staggering quantities that are being consumed, and the young ages at which these habits are being acquired. To my ethnobotanically trained clinical eye, this deluge of products appears to have been formulated primarily by opportunistic entrepreneurs.

As if vicariously partaking in the collective cerebral euphoria, I began having epiphanies. Is this veritable fountain of toxic stimulants at the root of the palpable epidemic of aggressive social behavior? Is this the result of prohibition against more benign intoxicants and ceremonial traditions of entheogenic wisdom? Is it linked to gun violence? Is it connected to the masculine identity propagated by the media, which glorifies the military and athletic prowess? What are the medical consequences for the brain and mind, for sleep and attention, for the heart and circulation, the glandular system, the teeth? What happens when these substances are mixed with alcohol, with prescription drugs? And most importantly, which ones should I try?

Suddenly, the deadline was upon me, and the Medicines From the Earth conference was looming. So many stimulants, so little time: which one would help me get this article finished, with a minimal amount of teeth grinding and residual darkness around the eyes?

I considered the immensity of the undertaking I had committed myself to, and went downstairs to make a cup of tea.

The Healthy Use of Stimulants

When discussing herbal stimulants, it is important to clarify exactly what the term means. In a fundamental way, as defined by classical systems such Chinese and Ayurvedic medicine as well as Western traditions such as the Physiomedicalists, all herbs are used for the two primary purposes of stimulating (warming) or relaxing (cooling). In reality, most have dual functions, such as the adaptogens that increase vitality while reducing stress, or aromatic herbs that stimulate digestive secretions while relaxing intestinal spasms. At the biochemical level the effects become even more complex. Even in the caffeine-containing herbs that are generally thought of as stimulants such as tea, there are compounds like theanine that have relaxant functions.

The first section of this article will be devoted to two herbs that are at the further end of the stimulant spectrum, guarana and yerba mate. These two species are representative of herbal stimulants in general, which are used both in traditional and contemporary society and have both numerous benefits and disadvantages; more importantly, these are probably the two most widely consumed herbal stimulants other than tea and coffee, and are now associated with new dangers because of their use and abuse in popular unregulated products. Coffee and tea will be mentioned briefly, but more importantly a section is dedicated to the dangers of concentrated stimulants such as "energy drinks" and other metabolic stimulants, as these represent a more important public health concern than the rather benign plant sources they are extracted from.

In general, our culture needs nutrition and relaxants far more than it needs stimulants. Even more importantly, it needs knowledge of how of to use all types of plants wisely. Stimulants, of all the classes of herbs, have been commercialized and abused the most by modern society. The overuse and misuse of these plants and preparations made from them is due partly to normal human cravings for more energy but also symptomatic of deeper malaises: the cumulative physical exhaustion, mental overstimulation and spiritual vacuity of our times.

Most of the herbal stimulants that have a long history of traditional use have many health benefits, even though they may contain primarily various forms and amounts of caffeine compounds. Like all herbs, there are dosages that are safe for long-term consumption, and dosages that can cause acute poisoning. Furthermore, there are individual constitutional differences that can dramatically affect the results of using a specific stimulant, as well as complex factors such as stress levels, blood sugar stability, cardiac health, diet and so on. For example, guarana that is traditionally prepared and consumed by Amazonian elders in their native environment probably produces a different effect than an energy drink containing guarana that is consumed by a stressed and exhausted person working three jobs in an urban environment.

One system that can help guide the use of stimulants is the Ayurvedic classification of vata, pitta, and kapha. A greatly simplified approach would say that the heavier, metabolically slower kapha types would benefit the most from herbal stimulants, while the already nervous and depleted vata type will be the most prone to overstimulation. This is an important consideration when reading studies that support the use of caffeine-containing herbs or products for fatigue, improved cognitive function, depression and so on, as those may be beneficial for one person but worsen conditions for another. There are not only great differences between individuals in their responses to stimulants, but in their tendencies for habituation, addiction and intensity of withdrawal as well.

Most importantly, people need to be educated about the causes of their symptoms, and become sensitive to whether or not the benefits of a moderate intake of stimulants outweighs the disadvantages. In my clinical practice, I am always amazed at how little awareness people have about the links between their habits and their symptoms. The true level of fatigue that people are medicating with stimulants often comes as a surprise when they attempt to eliminate them.

Clinically, there are rarely times when one needs to prescribe herbal stimulants, as the vast majority of patients need to relax and loosen their relationship with stimulant habituations and rejuvenate core vitality instead. The knowledge of stimulants is extremely useful, however, because herbal alternatives to coffee and low quality products can serve as a bridge to better self-management of stimulant overuse and stress in general, as stimulants are almost always used to support an overworked lifestyle or to push the body and mind to perform at the expense of sleep and cumulative nutrient and immune deficits.

Over the years of treating thousands of people for basically the same over-stimulation/exhaustion syndrome, I lost interest in propounding dogmatic health regimes, and gradually began suggesting commonsense lifestyle advice about stimulant use; part of this was because of my own growing appreciation for the cognitive enhancing properties of caffeine as I began doing more arduous writing. Instead of telling people to just quit coffee and then hear their tales of acute withdrawal while in Los Angeles traffic, I began advising a healthier relationship with their substances of choice, since the reality is that stimulants are almost a necessary part of life for many people.

The approach I advocate is both quantitative and qualitative: a smaller amount of a higher quality stimulant, enjoyed mindfully, is much healthier and more functional than a larger amount of lower quality stimulant used mindlessly. Another principle is to not try and be perfect in an insane world, but to reduce stimulant addiction to a manageable level, which is "take it or leave it" without causing a big metabolic upheaval. These have been my personal guiding principles for my own stimulant intake ever since, more or less.

Guarana (Paullinia cupana)

Guarana is a famous herbal stimulant native to the Amazon basin. It is a climbing plant of the maple family that is best known for its seeds, which are rich in guaranine, a compound of the caffeine family; the seeds contain around twice the amount of guaranine as caffeine in coffee beans, as well as smaller quantities of theophylline, theobromine and polyphenols.

Understanding guarana is important for two reasons: it is not a major medicine but has health benefits if used correctly, but it is also associated with serious medical incidents from excessive intake, mostly in energy drinks and weight loss products.

I have had some personal experience with guarana, in Brazil where it is widely consumed. My observation was that it is a relatively potent stimulant, more so than coffee. I suspect that there is a big difference in quality and effect between seeds prepared according to indigenous customs in Amazonian villages and commercially prepared powders, extracts and consumer products such as sodas. I would postulate that the more traditional the preparation, the richer the guarana is in compounds other than guaranine and therefore more therapeutic, while the more processed it becomes the more it is reduced to its caffeine-like compounds and utilized purely for stimulation.

Benefits

Protection Against Metabolic Diseases

There are numerous studies documenting the benefits of guarana. One of the more interesting of these was a study of 637 Amazonian elders, which found that those who habitually consumed guarana had lower rates of hypertension, obesity and metabolic syndrome (factors increasing the risk of cardiovascular disease and diabetes) than those who did not. (1)

This study was followed by another which found that those elderly who habitually ingested guarana had lower levels of low-density lipoprotein (LDL, "bad cholesterol") than those who did not consume it, validating its protective effects against cardiovascular disease. These lower levels were associated with guarana's polyphenol compounds and high antioxidant activity. (2)

Improved Cognitive Function

Guarana has been shown to improve cognitive functions, specifically attention, at low doses, both alone and in combination with ginseng. Because of its effectiveness at low doses, it is hypothesized that its actions are not based entirely on its caffeine compounds. (3)

Guarana, when given with a vitamin drink, has also been found to increase the speed and accuracy of mental tasks, and to reduce the mental fatigue associated with extended mental work. (4)

Reducing Fatigue

Guarana has been found effective for reducing fatigue in breast cancer patients undergoing chemotherapy, without affecting sleep quality or producing adverse reactions. (5)

Increased Endurance

Long term feeding (100 – 200 days) of guarana to mice significantly increased their physical endurance when subjected to stress; it also improves the memory of rats. (6)

Reducing Dental Plaque

The extract of guarana was found to have antibacterial properties against Staphylococcus mutans, and would therefore be useful against dental plaque and its associated symptoms. (7)

Anti-cancer Effects

Guarana is being studied for its anti-cancer potential. It has been found to "decrease proliferation and increase apoptosis of tumor cells, consequently reducing the tumor burden area" of melanoma lung metastases in mice. (8)

Guarana has been found to have anti-proliferative effects against other carcinomas as well. (9)

Appetite Suppression and Weight Loss

I am putting this section between "benefits" and "disadvantages," as it falls into both, depending on how it is used. Unfortunately, the commercialization of energy and weight loss products moves guarana out of its more benign role in traditional cultures into a more potentially dangerous role in modern usage.

Guarana has been found to have significant appetite suppressing effects, especially when combined with other stimulants such as yerba mate and damiana. (10)

The same combination of herbs was found to significantly delay gastric emptying, reduce the time to perceived gastric fullness and induce significant weight loss; its primary mode of action is significantly modulating gastric emptying. (11)

Disadvantages

The disadvantages of guarana stem from its commercialization and misuse in energy and weight loss products. While it probably won't have the same fate as ephedra, it is already getting some negative reports related to neurological and cardiac overstimulation. A case is reported of a healthy thirty-eight year old female who developed seizures after starting a supplement containing guarana, the seizures stopped after discontinuing the product. (12)

The ingredient list of this supplement sounds as if an enterprising individual simply mixed the most potent herbal simulants available: yerba mate, caffeine, guarana, damiana, green tea, ginseng, maca, and kola nut. (13)

Another thermogenic weight loss product based on caffeine and guarana was implicated in a case of hypertensive urgency, which was alleviated after discontinuing the product. Synephrine, a standardized form of bitter orange that is known to raise arterial pressure, was also an ingredient in this formula. (14)

Yerba Mate (Ilex paraguariensis)

I have more personal experience with this stimulant than with guarana; I met it originally in Brazil where it is widely consumed on a daily basis, probably more than guarana, and have continued my relationship with it intermittently. My impression of mate is that it is overall more nourishing and less stimulating than coffee and guarana, due to its lower levels of caffeine and rich antioxidant content, but there are many variables in the quality of the tea depending on whether the tree is grown in sun or shade and how it is processed.

Mate offers some interesting benefits and also has some significant disadvantages. It is an important herb for regulating lipid metabolism, and there is evidence that it has some protective effects against some cancers; paradoxically, it is also implicated as a causative factor in other cancers, mostly because of variables in how it is processed and consumed.

Benefits

Yerba mate has numerous health benefits besides its obvious use as a beverage for physical and mental energy.

Lipid Lowering

Mate tea has been found to lower serum triglycerides, low-density lipoprotein cholesterol concentrations and liver lipid levels, and suppress weight gain caused by a high fat diet. (15)

Mate tea has also been found to significantly reduce total body weight and lower serum levels of total cholesterol, triglyceride, and LDL, and elevate serum levels of high-density lipoprotein cholesterol, superoxide dismutase and gluta-thione peroxidase. Mate tea significantly ameliorated severe fatty degeneration of liver cells that occurred in the hyperlipidemic animals being studied. (16)

Mate's lipid lowering effects are attributed to phenolic compounds, which have potential application for cardiovascular disease. (17)

Anti-obesity

When obese mice were treated with yerba mate it produced a "marked atten-uation of weight gain, adiposity, a decrease in epididymal fat, and restoration of the serum levels of cholesterol, triglycerides, LDL cholesterol, and glucose. Additionally, it had a modulatory effect on the expression of several genes re-lated to obesity. (18)

A subsequent study suggests that mate may induce anorexic effects by di-rect induction of satiety and by stimulation of glucagon-like peptide 1 secre-tion and modulation of serum leptin levels. (19)

Anti-inflammatory

Another study suggests that the use of yerba mate extract may be useful for reducing low-grade inflammation associated with obesity. (20)

Yerba mate tea is proposed to have antioxidant and anti-inflammatory properties that could treat acute lung inflammation associated with exposure to cigarette smoke. (21)

Anti-herpes

Yerba mate was found to have in vitro anti-herpes effects by reducing infec-tivity through entry of the virus into cells, and spreading of virus from cell to cell. (22)

Anti-fungal

Water extract of yerba mate has been found to have anti-fungal action compa-rable to ketoconazole. (23)

Higher Bone Density

Postmenopausal women who drank at least one liter of yerba mate tea per day during the last four years or more were found to have greater bone mineral density than women who did not. (24)

Protective Against Cancer

Regular ingestion of yerba mate tea by mice increased resistance to DNA damage. Its mechanism is thought to be its abundance of free radical scavenging compounds. (25)

Disadvantages

Links to Cancer

The primary disadvantage with yerba mate is its suspected link as a causative factor to cancer, specifically esophageal squamous cell carcinoma; there are high rates of this type of cancer in the southern part of South America where mate is habitually consumed in larger amounts, and it is estimated that up to twenty percent may be associated with mate consumption. (26)

There are two primary factors associated with this risk, both of which can be controlled by the method of ingestion and the quality of tea that is purchased. The first is habitual intake of very hot mate, which has a higher risk than habitual intake of warm to cool mate. The second is the presence of carcinogenic compounds, which appear to be associated with the stages of processing the leaves.

The first factor is the amount of mate consumed, with higher amounts considered more of a risk factor than lower amounts. (27)

Drinking more than one liter per day is considered a risk factor, and drinking it very hot increases the risk two-fold. Drinking warm to cool mate along with alcohol and tobacco use increased the risk further, but drinking very hot mate along with alcohol and tobacco increased risk to maximum levels. (28)

Other beverages consumed at very hot temperatures are also associated with increased risk of esophageal cancer, so it is assumed that the carcinogenic effect is due to chronic thermal injury in the esophagus. (29)

It is postulated that drinking very hot mate could damage the mucosa or accelerate metabolic reactions with carcinogenic substances in tobacco and alcohol. (30)

According to another study, drinking cold mate does not increase the risk of cancer. (31)

Foods that are considered probable risk factors for prostate cancer included meat, milk, eggs, and mate consumption. (32)

It would appear from the above series of studies that the solution to the risk factors is to avoid drinking large amounts of very hot mate; however, another series of studies points to a new culprit that is not dependent on temperature of the drink. In these studies, the leaves of yerba mate were found to contain high levels of carcinogenic polycyclic aromatic hydrocarbons (PAHs), in both hot and cold infusions. (33)

The high levels of PAHs found in mate were attributed to degradation of compounds in the leaves during curing, specifically in the final stages where it undergoes rapid drying with wood fire. (34)

The lowest levels of PAH's were found in leaves that were not exposed to smoke in the drying process, indicating that the "smoked" varieties of mate on the market are to be avoided and that improved processing methods could further reduce the cancer risk. (35)

Quality Control

Another disadvantage of yerba mate is that most of the commercial brands consumed in South America have been found to have significant levels of fungal contamination. This may not be the case in the brands of tea that are now on the market in the US, especially those marketed as higher quality organic products, and regulations are probably more stringent than in Paraguay. (36)

Coffee and Tea

An immense amount of research and writing has been devoted to the subject of coffee and tea, so these favorite stimulants do not need to be covered here. However, I will mention a few points that I feel are relevant from my personal and clinical experience.

Drinking high quality organically cultivated coffee and tea are far less detrimental to the digestive, nervous and glandular systems than low-grade products, and have superior flavor as well.

Black teas tend to be more drying and acidic than green teas; the most biocompatible forms of tea, at least for me personally, are high-grade matcha and pu erh.

Tragically, many of the tea growing regions of Japan are in close proximity to the Fukushima nuclear plant.

People who are more physically active tend to tolerate the influence of caffeine from coffee and tea better than those who are not.

People who are under stress are affected more adversely by caffeine stimulation than those who are not. The most enjoyable way to imbibe caffeine is under relaxed conditions.

Drinking coffee and tea on an empty stomach, a very European habit, increases the likelihood of digestive symptoms, blood sugar imbalances and nervous tension. A small amount taken after a meal is tolerated better.

The less frequently tea and coffee are consumed, the more stimulating they tend to be. Over time, as people become habituated to caffeine, its stimulant effects decline.

Energy Drinks

Traditional herbal stimulants such as tea and mate pale in comparison to the new generation of energy drinks. Hundreds of new brands are appearing every year, literally one or more per day worldwide, and are available at every market, convenience store and gas station across the country. This relatively new phenomenon is a tidal wave of pink and blue sugar water loaded with caffeine, spiked with additional mate and guarana, topped off with a negligible dose of vitamins and amino acids, then marketed primarily to twenty year olds and teens. (37)

The data available on energy drinks closely parallels the information on weight loss products and "metabolism boosters." While there are more varieties of herbal and synthetic ingredients found in these two classes of products than energy drinks in general, the similarity is that, predictably, a majority of them are based on almost the same combination of ingredients. A quick perusal reveals that the most common herbal ingredients are green coffee extract, green tea, yerba mate, kola nut, the ubiquitous synthetic caffeine, and in many cases yohimbine alkaloids; it is therefore not surprising that many of the adverse reactions are also similar. Therefore, metabolic stimulant and weight loss products can be included in this discussion about the benefits and disadvantages of energy drinks.

Energy drinks are multi-billion dollar industry, with up to fifty percent of adolescents and young adults reporting use. (38)

Needless to say, emergency rooms have seen a sharp increase in visits for nausea, vomiting, heart palpitations and worse in those who unknowingly ingested hundreds of milligrams of pure caffeine, more caffeine from the herbal ingredients, and a dozen or more teaspoons of sugar, which can be easily done drinking two cans. Thousands of cases of acute caffeine intoxication happen annually, with just under half being teenagers. The risk of adverse reaction is higher in those with underlying medical problems such as diabetes, cardiac abnormalities, mood or behavioral disorders, or those on medications. (38)

Several cases of seizures caused by energy drinks have been reported. (39)

Besides the neurological and cardiac problems caused by caffeine, energy drinks destroy tooth enamel at higher rates than sports drinks, which probably destroy it faster than tea or mate. (40)

An even more serious problem is combining energy drinks with alcohol, which gives the illusion that one is more alert and less drunk, but in actuality the alcohol intoxication is undiminished; the subjective perception of intoxication is less, but the objective measures of coordination and visual reaction time are not. (41)

A high percentage of young people report consuming energy drinks with alcohol, a practice that has been confirmed creates higher rates of serious alcohol-related consequences. (41)

Those who consume higher amounts of energy drinks have also been found to drink alcohol more frequently and in higher quantities, with weekly or daily consumption strongly associated with alcohol dependency. (42)

Considering the availability of milder herbal stimulants with less overall caffeine and more holistic health benefits, it would be easy to say that energy drinks have no benefits and instead have only moderate to serious disadvantages. However, the reality is that consuming sugar water with caffeine increases people's energy and improves their cognitive functions, specifically mental concentration...thus the popularity. (43)(44)

Of course, it is not just glucose or caffeine by themselves that do the trick, but their synergistic effect is even greater; in the astute words of a report in Psychopharmacology: "These data suggest that there is some degree of synergy between the cognition-modulating effects of glucose and caffeine which merits further investigation." (45)

Besides the attraction to mental stimulants in college students, those who drive a lot are also prime candidates for stimulant consumption, with the associated benefits of increased alertness on long drives. (46)

Athletes are also prime targets of marketing campaigns. While there is evidence that energy drinks improve reaction time, energy, and mental focus, they are also associated with gastrointestinal symptoms, cardiac arrhythmia, blood pressure increases, potential effects on lipids and blood glucose, seizures and heart attack. (47) (48)

Energy drinks appear to increase pain tolerance, another desirable attraction for athletes. (49)

It is not surprising to discover that there is a psychological term for a type of male that is typically attracted to energy drinks: "toxic jock." The strength of jock identity has been correlated with frequency of energy drink consumption. (50)

While the identity of being an "athlete" is linked with improved mental and social wellbeing, the opposite is true of the "jock" identity, which is linked with the opposite, including higher risk of suicide. (51)

Caffeine Addiction and Withdrawal

Many people are surprised to discover they have a caffeine addiction. I have been surprised to see people going through the classic withdrawal symptoms of headache, grogginess, depression, and digestive disturbance without associating the fact that they had not had their normal caffeine intake. The best diagnostic method to determine if the symptoms are related to caffeine withdrawal is a shot of espresso.

The biochemistry of caffeine addiction and withdrawal is too large a topic for this paper, but we should not conclude without some discussion of how to assist patients through the process.

It is easier to end a substantial caffeine addiction if one eats a healthy diet that is rich in phytonutrients for a period of time first. Stopping coffee while continuing with a poor quality diet is more difficult; processed foods, sugars and often gluten lower vitality and increase cravings for caffeine.

Drinking water helps lessen caffeine withdrawal; drinking alcohol worsens it.

It is easier to stop suddenly if one is able to take time off from work and not required to maintain normal physical and mental energy levels. If not, it is easier to transition gradually and to substitute green tea and mate for coffee.

Fresh air and gentle exercise can help alleviate symptoms.

There are many herbs that can be helpful at reducing the length and severity of caffeine withdrawal symptoms. Strong infusions of aromatics such as peppermint, rosemary, and tulsi are good; relaxants such as chamomile, lavender and lemon balm may work well for some; the essential oils from all of these could be beneficial for aromatherapy purposes. Anti-spasmotics such as California poppy could be considered. The milder adaptogens that also have relaxant effects such as ashwagandha may be helpful, as well as the ginsengs, specifically American.

Acupuncture and massage are helpful.

Conclusion

Since caffeine is the underlying theme that runs throughout the subject of stimulants, it would be fitting to conclude with a description of its actions from King's American Dispensatory: "Mental activity is pronounced, thought is rapid, and so great is the cerebral stimulation that an enormous amount of brain power is developed, so that individuals are capable of prolonged and severe mental application. The reasoning faculties are sharpened, and there is also a marked capacity for physical labor."

References

(1) Phytother Res. 2011 Feb 22. doi: 10.1002/ptr.3437. [Epub ahead of print]

Habitual Intake of Guaraná and Metabolic Morbidities: An Epidemiological Study of an Elderly Amazonian Population. Costa Krewer C, Ribeiro EE, Ribeiro EA, Moresco RN, Ugalde Marques da Rocha MI, Santos Montagner GF, Machado MM, Viegas K, Brito E, Cruz IB. Departamento de Morfologia, Centro de Ciências da Saúde, Universidade Federal de Santa Maria, Brazil; Programa de Pós-Graduação em Bioquímica Toxicológica, Centro de Ciências Naturais e Exatas, Universidade Federal de Santa Maria, Brazil.

(2) Lipids Health Dis. 2013 Feb 8;12:12. Guaraná (Paullinia cupana Kunth) effects on LDL oxidation in elderly people: an in vitro and in vivo study. Portella Rde L, Barcelos RP, da Rosa EJ, Ribeiro EE, da Cruz IB, Suleiman L, Soares FA. Departamento de Química, Centro de Ciências Naturais e Exatas, Universidade Federal de Santa Maria, Campus UFSM, Santa Maria, RS, Brazil.

(3) Pharmacol Biochem Behav. 2004 Nov;79(3):401-11. Improved cognitive performance in human volunteers following administration of guarana (Paullinia cupana) extract: comparison and interaction with Panax ginseng. Kennedy DO, Haskell CF, Wesnes KA, Scholey AB.

Human Cognitive Neuroscience Unit, Division of Psychology, Northumbria University, Newcastle upon Tyne, NE1 8ST, United Kingdom.

(4) Appetite. 2008 Mar-May;50(2-3):506-13. Epub 2007 Oct 30. Improved cognitive performance and mental fatigue following a multi-vitamin and mineral supplement with added guaraná (Paullinia cupana).

Kennedy DO, Haskell CF, Robertson B, Reay J, Brewster-Maund C, Luedemann J, Maggini S, Ruf M, Zangara A, Scholey AB. Human Cognitive Neuroscience Unit, Northumbria University, Newcastle upon Tyne NE1 8ST, UK.

(5) J Altern Complement Med. 2011 Jun;17(6):505-12. doi: 10.1089/acm.2010.0571. Epub 2011 May 25.

Guarana (Paullinia cupana) improves fatigue in breast cancer patients undergoing systemic chemotherapy.

de Oliveira Campos MP, Riechelmann R, Martins LC, Hassan BJ, Casa FB, Del Giglio A.

Department of Hematology/Oncology, ABC School of Medicine, Santo André, Sao Paulo, Brazil .

(6) J Ethnopharmacol. 1997 Feb;55(3):223-9. Pharmacological activity of Guarana (Paullinia cupana Mart.) in laboratory animals. Espinola EB, Dias RF, Mattei R, Carlini EA.

Laboratório de Tecnologia Farmacêutica, Universidade Federal da Paraíba, Brazil.

(7) Molecules. 2007 Aug 20;12(8):1950-63. Antioxidant capacity and in vitro prevention of dental plaque formation by extracts and condensed tannins of Paullinia cupana.

Yamaguti-Sasaki E, Ito LA, Canteli VC, Ushirobira TM, Ueda-Nakamura T, Dias Filho BP, Nakamura CV, de Mello JC. Programa de Pós-Graduação em Ciências Farmacêuticas, Universidade Estadual de Maringá, Av. Colombo, 5790, BR-87020-900, Maringá, PR, Brazil.

(8) Braz J Med Biol Res. 2008 Apr;41(4):305-10. Paullinia cupana Mart var. sorbilis, guaraná, reduces cell proliferation and increases apoptosis of B16/F10 melanoma lung metastases in mice.

Fukumasu H, Avanzo JL, Nagamine MK, Barbuto JA, Rao KV, Dagli ML.

Laboratório de Oncologia Experimental e Comparada, Departamento de Patologia, Faculdade de Medicina Veterinária e Zootecnia, Universidade de São Paulo, São Paulo, SP, Brasil.

(9) Phytother Res. 2011 Jan;25(1):11-6. doi: 10.1002/ptr.3216. Paullinia cupana Mart. var. sorbilis, guarana, increases survival of Ehrlich ascites carcinoma (EAC) bearing mice by decreasing cyclin-D1 expression and inducing a G0/G1 cell cycle arrest in EAC cells.

Fukumasu H, Latorre AO, Zaidan-Dagli ML. Department of Pathology, School of Veterinary Medicine and Animal Sciences, University of São Paulo, São Paulo, SP, Brazil.

(10) Appetite. 2013 Mar;62:84-90. doi: 10.1016/j.appet.2012.11.018. Epub 2012 Dec 1.

Acute effects of a herb extract formulation and inulin fibre on appetite, energy intake and food choice.

Harrold JA, Hughes GM, O'Shiel K, Quinn E, Boyland EJ, Williams NJ, Halford JC.

Kissileff Laboratory for the Study of Human Ingestive Behaviour, Department of Experimental Psychology, Institute of Psychology, Health and Society, University of Liverpool, Eleanor Rathbone Building, Bedford Street South, Liverpool L69 7ZA, UK.

(11) J Hum Nutr Diet. 2001 Jun;14(3):243-50. Weight loss and delayed gastric emptying following a South American herbal preparation in overweight patients. Andersen T, Fogh J.

Department of Ultrasound, Medical Center Charlottenlund, Trunnevangen 4A, DK 2920, Charlottenlund, Denmark.

(12) J Diet Suppl. 2013 Mar;10(1):1-5. doi: 10.3109/19390211.2012.758215. Epub 2013 Feb 4.

Potential toxicity of caffeine when used as a dietary supplement for weight loss.

Pendleton M, Brown S, Thomas CM, Odle B. 1Baptist Medical Center, Wake Forest University , Winston-Salem , United States.

(13) http://dietarysupplements.nlm.nih.gov/dietary/detail.jsp?contain=26003001&name=Zantrex-3&pageD=brand

(14) J Pharm Pract. 2011 Jun 6. Hypertensive Urgency Associated With Xenadrine EFX Use.

Moaddeb J, Tofade TS, Bevins MB.

(15) Obesity (Silver Spring). 2010 Jan;18(1):42-7. doi: 10.1038/oby.2009.189. Epub 2009 Jun 18.

Maté tea inhibits in vitro pancreatic lipase activity and has hypolipidemic effect on high-fat diet-induced obese mice.

Martins F, Noso TM, Porto VB, Curiel A, Gambero A, Bastos DH, Ribeiro ML, Carvalho Pde O. São Francisco University, Bragança Paulista, Brazil.

(16) Phytother Res. 2012 Oct 10. doi: 10.1002/ptr.4856. [Epub ahead of print]

Aqueous Extract of Yerba Mate Tea Lowers Atherosclerotic Risk Factors in a Rat Hyperlipidemia Model.

Gao H, Liu Z, Wan W, Qu X, Chen M.

College of Pharmacy, Taishan Medical University, Taian, 271016, PR, China.

(17) <u>Fitoterapia.</u> 2013 Feb 17;86C:115-122. doi: 10.1016/j.fito-te.2013.02.008.

Lipid-lowering effects of standardized extracts of Ilex paraguariensis in high-fat-diet rats.

<u>Balzan S, Hernandes A, Reichert CL, Donaduzzi C, Pires VA, Gasparotto A Junior, Cardozo EL Junior.</u>

Instituto de Ciências Biológicas, Médicas e da Saúde, Universidade Paranaense, Toledo, PR, Brazil.

(18) <u>Obesity (Silver Spring).</u> 2009 Dec;17(12):2127-33. doi: 10.1038/oby.2009.158. Epub 2009 May 14.

Antiobesity effects of yerba maté extract (Ilex paraguariensis) in high-fat diet-induced obese mice.

<u>Arçari DP, Bartchewsky W, dos Santos TW, Oliveira KA, Funck A, Pedrazzoli J, de Souza MF, Saad MJ, Bastos DH, Gambero A, Carvalho Pde O, Ribeiro ML.</u>

Unidade Integrada de Farmacologia e Gastroenterologia, Universidade São Francisco, Bragança Paulista, Brazil.

(19) <u>Biol Pharm Bull.</u> 2011;34(12):1849-55. Mate tea (Ilex paraguariensis) promotes satiety and body weight lowering in mice: involvement of glucagon-like peptide-1.

<u>Hussein GM, Matsuda H, Nakamura S, Hamao M, Akiyama T, Tamura K, Yoshikawa M.</u> Kyoto Pharmaceutical University, Japan.

(20) <u>J Nutr Biochem.</u> 2012 Jul 25. [Epub ahead of print] Yerba mate extract (Ilex paraguariensis) attenuates both central and peripheral inflammatory effects of diet-induced obesity in rats.

<u>Pimentel GD, Lira FS, Rosa JC, Caris AV, Pinheiro F, Ribeiro EB, Oller do Nascimento CM, Oyama LM.</u>

(21) <u>Nutrition.</u> 2008 Apr;24(4):375-81. doi: 10.1016/j.nut.2008.01.002. Epub 2008 Feb 20.

Mate tea reduced acute lung inflammation in mice exposed to cigarette smoke.

<u>Lanzetti M, Bezerra FS, Romana-Souza B, Brando-Lima AC, Koatz VL, Porto LC, Valenca SS.</u>

Tissue Repair Laboratory, Histology and Embryology Department, Roberto

Alcântara Gomes Institute of Biology, Rio de Janeiro State University, Rio de Janeiro, Brazil.

(22) Phytother Res. 2012 Apr;26(4):535-40. doi: 10.1002/ptr.3590. Epub 2011 Sep 14.

Effects of Ilex paraguariensis A. St. Hil. (yerba mate) on herpes simplex virus types 1 and 2 replication.

Lückemeyer DD, Müller VD, Moritz MI, Stoco PH, Schenkel EP, Barardi CR, Reginatto FH, Simões CM.

Department of Pharmaceutical Sciences, Universidade Federal de Santa Catarina, UFSC, Florianópolis, SC, Brazil.

(23) Phytother Res. 2010 May;24(5):715-9. doi: 10.1002/ptr.3004. Antifungal activity of the aqueous extract of Ilex paraguariensis against Malassezia furfur. Filip R, Davicino R, Anesini C.

Instituto de Química y Metabolismo del Fármaco (IQUIME-FA-UBA-CONICET), University of Buenos Aires, Buenos Aires, Argentina.

(24) Bone. 2012 Jan;50(1):9-13. doi: 10.1016/j.bone.2011.08.029. Epub 2011 Sep 3.

Yerba Mate (Ilex paraguariensis) consumption is associated with higher bone mineral density in postmenopausal women. Conforti AS, Gallo ME, Saraví FD.

Program for the Prevention and Treatment of Osteoporosis, Obra Social de Empleados Públicos, Mendoza, Argentina.

(25) Protective effects of mate tea (Ilex paraguariensis) on H2O2-induced DNA damage and DNA repair in mice. Miranda DD, Arçari DP, Pedrazzoli J Jr, Carvalho Pde O, Cerutti SM, Bastos DH, Ribeiro ML.

Unidade Integrada de Farmacologia e Gastroenterologia, Universidade São Francisco, Av. São Francisco de Assis, 218. Jd. São José, Bragança Paulista, SP, Brazil.

(26) Epidemiology. 1994 Nov;5(6):583-90. Maté, coffee, and tea consumption and risk of cancers of the upper aerodigestive tract in southern Brazil. Pintos J, Franco EL, Oliveira BV, Kowalski LP, Curado MP, Dewar R. Department of Epidemiology, Armand-Frappier Institute, Goiania, Brazil.

(27) Mutagenesis. 2008 Jul;23(4):261-5. doi: 10.1093/mutage/gen011. Epub 2008 Feb 27.

Dis Esophagus. 2012 Aug 14. doi: 10.1111/j.1442-2050.2012.01393.x. [Epub ahead of print]

Maté consumption and the risk of esophageal squamous cell carcinoma: a meta-analysis.

Andrici J, Eslick GD. The Whiteley-Martin Research Centre, The Discipline of Surgery, The University of Sydney, Sydney Medical School, Nepean, Penrith, New South Wales, Australia.

(28) Cancer Epidemiol Biomarkers Prev. 2003 Jun;12(6):508-13. Maté consumption and the risk of squamous cell esophageal cancer in uruguay. Sewram V, De Stefani E, Brennan P, Boffetta P.

Promec Unit, Medical Research Council, Tygerberg, South Africa.

(29) Int J Cancer. 2000 Nov 15;88(4):658-64. Influence of mate drinking, hot beverages and diet on esophageal cancer risk in South America. Castellsagué X, Muñoz N, De Stefani E, Victora CG, Castelletto R, Rolón PA. Servei d'Epidemiologia i Registre del Càncer, Institut Català d'Oncologia, L'Hospitalet de Llobregat, Barcelona, Spain. xcastellsague@ico.scs.ed

(30) Rev Panam Salud Publica. 2009 Jun;25(6):530-9. Cancer and yerba mate consumption: a review of possible associations. Loria D, Barrios E, Zanetti R. Instituto de Oncología "Angel H. Roffo," Buenos Aires, Argentina.

(31) Cancer Epidemiol Biomarkers Prev. 1995 Sep;4(6):595-605. Hot and cold mate drinking and esophageal cancer in Paraguay. Rolón PA, Castellsagué X, Benz M, Muñoz N.

Laboratorio de Anatomia Patológica y Citología, Asunción, Paraguay.

(32) Cancer Causes Control. 2012 Jul;23(7):1031-8. doi: 10.1007/s10552-012-9968-z. Epub 2012 Apr 28.

Food groups and risk of prostate cancer: a case-control study in Uruguay.

Deneo-Pellegrini H, Ronco AL, De Stefani E, Boffetta P, Correa P, Mendilaharsu M, Acosta G.

Grupo de Epidemiología, Departamento de Anatomía Patológica, Hospital de Clínicas, Universidad de la República, Montevideo, Uruguay.

(33) Cancer Epidemiol Biomarkers Prev. 2008 May;17(5):1262-8. doi: 10.1158/1055-9965.EPI-08-0025.

High levels of carcinogenic polycyclic aromatic hydrocarbons in mate drinks.

Kamangar F, Schantz MM, Abnet CC, Fagundes RB, Dawsey SM.

Division of Cancer Epidemiology and Genetics, National Cancer Institute,

Bethesda, MD, USA.

(34) Food Addit Contam Part A Chem Anal Control Expo Risk Assess. 2010 Jun;27(6):776-82. doi: 10.1080/19440041003587310. Occurrence of polycyclic aromatic hydrocarbons throughout the processing stages of erva-mate (Ilex paraguariensis). Vieira MA, Maraschin M, Rovaris AA, Amboni RD, Pagliosa CM, Xavier JJ, Amante ER. Department of Food Science and Technology, Federal University of Santa Catarina, 88034-001 Florianopolis, SC, Brazil.

(35) Environ Sci Technol. 2012 Dec 18;46(24):13488-93. doi: 10.1021/ es303494s. Epub 2012 Dec 3.

Significant variation in the concentration of carcinogenic polycyclic aromatic hydrocarbons in yerba maté samples by brand, batch, and processing method.

Golozar A, Fagundes RB, Etemadi A, Schantz MM, Kamangar F, Abnet CC, Dawsey SM.

Division of Cancer Epidemiology and Genetics, National Cancer Institute, Bethesda, Maryland, USA.

(36) Transpl Infect Dis. 2010 Dec;12(6):565-9. doi: 10.1111/j.1399-3062.2010.00554.x. Drinking yerba mate infusion: a potential risk factor for invasive fungal diseases? Vieira NO, Peres A, Aquino VR, Pasqualotto AC. Microbiology Laboratory, Centro Universitário Metodista IPA, Porto Alegre, Brazil.

(37) J Am Acad Nurse Pract. 2012 Feb;24(2):70-6. doi: 10.1111/j.1745-7599.2011.00689.x. Epub 2012 Jan 31. Energy drinks: what is all the hype? The dangers of energy drink consumption.

Rath M. University of Mary, Steele, North Dakota 58482, USA.

(38) Pediatrics. 2011 Mar;127(3):511-28. doi: 10.1542/peds.2009-3592. Epub 2011 Feb 14.

Health effects of energy drinks on children, adolescents, and young adults.

Seifert SM, Schaechter JL, Hershorin ER, Lipshultz SE. Department of Pediatrics and Pediatric Integrative Medicine Program, University of Miami, Leonard M. Miller School of Medicine, Miami, Florida 33101, USA.

(39) Epilepsy Behav. 2007 May;10(3):504-8. Epub 2007 Mar 8. New-onset seizures in adults: possible association with consumption of popular energy drinks. Iyadurai SJ, Chung SS.

Department of Neurology, Barrow Neurological Institute, St. Joseph's Hospital and Medical Center, Phoenix, AZ 58013, USA.

(40) <u>Gen Dent.</u> 2012 May-Jun;60(3):190-7; quiz 198-9. A comparison of sports and energy drinks—Physiochemical properties and enamel dissolution. <u>Jain P, Hall-May E, Golabek K, Agustin MZ.</u>

Department of Growth, Development, and Structure, Southern Illinois University School of Dental Medicine, Alton, Illinois, USA.

(41) <u>Arch Pediatr.</u> 2010 Nov;17(11):1625-31. doi: 10.1016/j. arcped.2010.08.001.

[Risks of energy drinks in youths]. <u>Bigard AX.</u> Institut de recherche biomédicale des armées, 24, avenue des Maquis-du-Grésivaudan, 38700 La Tronche cedex, France.

(42) <u>Alcohol Clin Exp Res.</u> 2011 Feb;35(2):365-75. doi: 10.1111/j.1530-0277.2010.01352.x. Epub 2010 Nov 12. Energy drink consumption and increased risk for alcohol dependence. <u>Arria AM, Caldeira KM, Kasperski SJ, Vincent KB, Griffiths RR, O'Grady KE.</u> Center on Young Adult Health and Development, Department of Family Science, University of Maryland School of Public Health, College Park, 20740, USA.

(43) <u>Exp Clin Psychopharmacol.</u> 2010 Dec;18(6):553-61. doi: 10.1037/a0021740. Acute effects of a glucose energy drink on behavioral control. <u>Howard MA, Marczinski CA.</u>

Department of Psychological Science, Northern Kentucky University, Highland Heights, KY 41099, USA.

(44) <u>Appetite.</u> 2004 Jun;42(3):331-3. A glucose-caffeine 'energy drink' ameliorates subjective and performance deficits during prolonged cognitive demand. <u>Kennedy DO, Scholey AB.</u>

Human Cognitive Neuroscience Unit, Division of Psychology, University of Northumbria, Newcastle upon Tyne, NE1 8ST, UK.

(45) <u>Psychopharmacology (Berl).</u> 2004 Nov;176(3-4):320-30. Epub 2004 Jul 31.Cognitive and physiological effects of an "energy drink": an evaluation of the whole drink and of glucose, caffeine and herbal flavouring fractions. <u>Scholey AB, Kennedy DO.</u> Human Cognitive Neuroscience Unit, Division of Psychology, Northumbria University, Newcastle upon Tyne, NE1 8ST, UK.

(46) <u>Psychopharmacology (Berl).</u> 2011 Apr;214(3):737-45. doi: 10.1007/s00213-010-2078-2. Epub 2010 Nov 10. Positive effects of Red Bull® Energy Drink on driving performance during prolonged driving.

Mets MA, Ketzer S, Blom C, van Gerven MH, van Willigenburg GM, Olivier B, Verster JC.

Division of Pharmacology, Utrecht Institute for Pharmaceutical Sciences, Utrecht University, P.O. Box 80082, 3508 TB, Utrecht, The Netherlands.

(47) Am J Health Syst Pharm. 2013 Apr 1;70(7):577-88. doi: 10.2146/ajhp120118.

Efficacy and safety of ingredients found in preworkout supplements. Eudy AE, Gordon LL, Hockaday BC, Lee DA, Lee V, Luu D, Martinez CA, Ambrose PJ. Anne E. Eudy is a student, Eshelman School of Pharmacy, University of North Carolina at Chapel Hill

(48) Phys Sportsmed. 2010 Jun;38(2):171-9. doi: 10.3810/psm.2010.06.1796. Energy drinks: a review of use and safety for athletes. Duchan E, Patel ND, Feucht C. Michigan State University, Kalamazoo Center for Medical Studies, Kalamazoo, MI.

(49) Amino Acids. 2010 Apr;38(4):1193-200. doi: 10.1007/s00726-009-0330-z. Epub 2009 Aug 4.

Effect of Red Bull energy drink on cardiovascular and renal function. Ragsdale FR, Gronli TD, Batool N, Haight N, Mehaffey A, McMahon EC, Nalli TW, Mannello CM, Sell CJ, McCann PJ, Kastello GM, Hooks T, Wilson T. Department of Biology, Winona State University, Winona, MN 55987, USA.

(50) J Am Coll Health. 2008 Mar-Apr;56(5):481-9. doi: 10.3200/JACH.56.5.481-490.

Wired: energy drinks, jock identity, masculine norms, and risk taking. Miller KE. University at Buffalo, Research Institute on Addictions, Buffalo, NY 14203, USA.

(51) Sociol Sport J. 2009 Jun 1;26(2):335-356. Mental Well-Being and Sport-Related Identities in College Students. Miller KE, Hoffman JH. University at Buffalo, Research Institute on Addictions, 1021 Main Street, Buffalo, NY, 14203.

V

Dental Health
Natural Approaches

Introduction

Botanical medicine offers many effective treatments for common dental problems and is probably the best modality, along with diet, for maintaining good
oral hygiene and preventing problems without using questionable ingredients.
Because of the strong link between chronic infection in the mouth and other
health conditions, and the known and unknown dangers of xenobiotic substances used in dental treatments, simple natural remedies should be viewed as
having not just local benefits but an important role in maintaining wellbeing
and reducing the need for dental procedures that can have long term adverse
immunological consequences. Additionally, if we compare the astronomical
costs of clinical dental care with the extremely low cost of most of the botanical ingredients used for oral hygiene, we can conclude that not only are these
remedies some of the most important for overall health but some of the most
cost effective as well.

The Major Dental Diseases

There are three primary dental diseases: tooth decay, gingivitis and periodontitis. There are diverse causes and multiple types of these conditions, but the
most widespread and common forms have a similar etiology and therefore
similar approaches using herbal treatment. While there are limitations to what
natural remedies can do once teeth and their root structures are damaged, botanical preparations can be remarkably effective at treating the inflammation
and infection underlying most symptoms, and are probably the best approach
for general prevention and maintaining good dental hygiene.

Tooth Decay

Tooth decay is as old as hominids; the incidence was low in aboriginal hunt-
ing and gathering societies, increased with the advent of agriculture and ap-

pearance of grains in the diet, and is now the world's most prevalent disease, followed by periodontitis; about 2.4 billion people worldwide have caries, or about 36 percent of the population.

The etiology of caries is the same as the major forms of gingivitis and periodontitis: bacterial infection with acidification from carbohydrate fermentation. In the case of tooth decay the acidification causes demineralization of the surface structures of the teeth.

Herbal preparations in conjunction with nutrition are probably the most important approach for preventing tooth decay. Minor lesions can remineralize and there is an abundance of botanical remedies for symptomatic treatment of toothaches, but after cavities are established they must be treated by conventional dentistry; because of the prevalence of toxic materials in dentistry, it is important to work with holistic practitioners who are trained in minimizing the impacts of these toxins.

Gingivitis

Gingivitis is inflammation of the gums. There are several types and causes; the most widespread is termed "plaque-induced," as it is caused by the bacterial biofilm of plaque and the immune system's response against it. Plaque induced gingivitis is subdivided into various types depending on the influence of other factors as systemic health, medications and nutrition. Other types of gingivitis can be caused by factors other than plaque, including other types of infection, trauma, and reactions to foreign substances such as dental materials.

The primary signs and symptoms of gingivitis are halitosis, swollen gums that can be red or purple, gum tenderness and pain, and bleeding gums.

The etiology of plaque-induced gingivitis is the same as caries: accumulation of the bacterial biofilm that produce acid toxins and enzymes; in this case it provokes inflammatory responses in the gum tissue.

The primary treatment for most cases of gingivitis is plaque removal. Because plaque is a bacterial biofilm, numerous botanical approaches in conjunction with mechanical cleansing are viable and effective.

Gingivitis is not destructive and does not necessarily progress to periodontitis, but periodontitis and the deeper tissue damage it causes is always preceded by gingivitis.

Periodontitis

Periodontitis is a group of inflammatory diseases that affect the four tissues of the periodontium: gums, cementum (outer layer of roots of teeth), alveolar bone, and periodontal ligaments that connect teeth to the alveolar bone. Like gingivitis, it is caused by the bacterial biofilm on the surface of the teeth and the immune system's response to it.

Periodontitis affects about 750 million people in the world, about ten percent of the population; in the U.S. its prevalence is up to fifty percent. The disease is classified into various categories according to severity and etiology, which includes gingivitis; several of these forms are considered destructive and irreversible.

Symptoms of periodontitis include gingivitis, bleeding gums, halitosis, metallic taste in mouth, receding gums, pockets between teeth and gums, and in the later stages loose teeth. Periodontitis can progress without pain or symptoms, and the condition can become advanced before it is discovered. Periodontitis increases inflammation in the body and has been linked to stroke, heart attack and atherosclerosis.

Periodontitis should be considered in the realm of conventional dental diagnosis and treatment, with botanical remedies offering many complementary and alternative approaches. Herbal medicine can play an important role in prevention of periodontitis through daily hygiene. There are many reports of successful botanical treatment of chronic and advanced cases using more intensive methods such as herbal packs for the gums, and treating loose teeth (one of the symptoms of advanced periodontitis) was a routine part of early American herbal practice.

Toxic Dental Products and Materials

While tooth decay, gingivitis and periodontitis are the three most important and widespread dental diseases, dental materials are increasingly implicated as causative factors in a number of immunological problems. In my clinical practice I have always considered the patient's dental history, and have found many suspected links between dental work and systemic problems, including deterioration of mercury fillings and thyroid function, root canals and onset of chronic sinus infections, use of plastics and resins and later onset of autoimmune disorders, and so on. Many of these are well established in the medical literature, such as the neurological problems caused by mercury exposure in the dental profession, immune reactions to resins and implants, and chronic infections around root canals; others are relatively new and have yet to receive attention.

In comparison to the numerous simple, nontoxic and effective botanical ingredients, the vast array of dental and oral care products available over the counter look suspiciously like ingenious ways of recycling toxic waste and finding new uses of chemical compounds. This long list includes various forms of fluoride; artificial colorings, flavorings and sweeteners; triclosan, an antibacterial and antifungal compound used in soaps that degrades into dioxins, poisons ecosystems and is a known endocrine disrupter; questionable substances that are Generally Recognized as Safe by the FDA such as propylene glycol; and numerous industrial cleansing agents such as trisodium phosphate, once used in toilet cleaners but now discontinued because it damages metal.

The list of materials used in dental procedures is more extensive: alloys of various metals, bone substitutes, resins, ceramics, cements, sealants, plastics, nylons, silicones, adhesives and more. The most famous of these is probably the mercury-based so-called "silver amalgams," which, in spite of their obvious and known toxicity to both humans and the environment are still in wide spread use. This arsenal of compounds is potentially more dangerous from the immunological standpoint than those found in toothpastes and mouthwashes, as the materials are implanted in the mouth and undoubtedly degrade and interact with other materials over time.

The impact of dental materials on overall health and the immune system is not the primary topic of this paper, but it illustrates the most important reason for becoming knowledgeable about botanical alternatives: when it comes to self care and preventive healthcare routines, there is probably nothing more basic and important that we can do than to avoid, unless absolutely necessary, the use of implanted dental materials. While much is known about the long-term effects of these substances, what is more important is what is not known.

One striking example that has emerged in recent years is Morgellons, sometimes referred to as "springtails." This bizarre condition is characterized by the emergence of thread-like exudates from persistent skin lesions, accompanied by intense sensations of insects crawling, biting and stinging. It has been proposed that this syndrome comes from new nanoparticles or GMO crops, while the medical community generally regards it as "delusional parasitosis."

While these hypotheses may be plausible, the explanation that I have found most convincing comes from Dr. Omar Amin, an expert parasitologist. He has renamed the disorder "Neuro-Cutaneous Syndrome," and attributes its cause to inflammation of peripheral nerves in response to dental xenobiotics. To sum up one of his many medical papers on the subject: "Components in the calcium hydroxide dental sealants Dycal, Life and Sealapex have been identified as the sources of the observed symptoms." (1)

Microbial Ecology

Maintaining oral health and treating common dental problems is fundamentally a process of regulating a complex microbial environment. This regulatory process is based partly on a diet that provides high quality nutrients and avoids frequent intake of carbohydrates and sugars, partly on routine cleansing, both mechanical and biological, and partly on maintaining and promoting healthy salivary flow; the primary objective is controlling bacterial overgrowth of pathogenic bacteria that are the cause of conditions such as caries, gingivitis, and periodontitis.

There are a wide variety of botanical species used in various forms for achieving these purposes, including chewing sticks, toothpowders containing herbal and mineral ingredients, and herbal and essential oil mouthwashes. Many of these are long-standing remedies in various cultures that are now being shown to be as effective or more than synthetic products. The effectiveness of these botanicals is generally based on the combination of their mechanical cleansing abilities combined with the presence of antimicrobial and anti-inflammatory compounds.

Streptococcus mutans

Historically, the prevalent model of tooth decay and conditions such as gingivitis has been based on a bacterial theory, with Streptococcus mutans being identified as the primary culprit. Microbes such as S. mutans in the biofilm of plaque cause caries and other infectious conditions though three mechanisms: their adhesive properties, their ability to create an acidic environment and their tolerance to that acidity. (2)

The role of a healthy bacterial ecology in the mouth and on the teeth is the same as that which colonizes the mucus membranes in general, which is to provide immunological protection against overgrowth of pathogenic species and acidification of the terrain this causes. It is known that when the teeth are colonized by healthy bacteria they are less likely to become colonized with pathogens such as S. mutans and the development of caries is less likely. Prevention and treatment of all the common oral and dental problems therefore entail the same strategies that are used in other conditions of the mucus membranes when they are inflamed and infected, which is controlling pathogens with antimicrobial and anti-inflammatory remedies while supporting the healthy microbial terrain, generally with mucilaginous herbs. (3)

While S. mutans is still considered to be the most important pathogen of the mouth, a more holistic model has emerged which views the processes of inflammation and infection at the root of these problems as an ecological problem caused by imbalances in the dynamic relationships among plaque causing microbes, dietary carbohydrates and sugars, saliva and pH levels in the mouth. Fermentable carbohydrates in the mouth cause an increase of pH by acidogenic microbes of the plaque biofilm; this acidification of the terrain increases when the antimicrobial and mechanical cleansing properties of saliva are diminished by reduced flow. (4)

Saliva

Saliva plays a crucial role in dental and oral health. Mechanically, its flow regulates exposure of tooth surfaces to carbohydrate fermentation and the microbial composition of plaque, thereby regulating overall pH of the mouth. (5)

Saliva contains compounds that inhibit bacterial fermentation and acidity that cause oral inflammation and infection. Enzymes such as amylase and salivary lipase start the digestion of starches and fats and reduce bacterial build-up on the teeth, supported by antibacterial agents as secretory IgA, and other compounds such as proline-rich proteins, which support formation of enamel.

Salivary flow is directly related to the pH of the mouth and surface of the teeth. There is a continual interplay between the flow of saliva and demineralization and remineralization on the surface of the teeth: when the flow of saliva decreases, the acidity levels of the mouth in general and on the teeth specifically increase.

Considering the importance of saliva for maintaining a healthy bacterial ecology of the mouth, it is not difficult to understand that there is a relationship between the quantity and quality of salivary flow and pH levels created by the acidic carbohydrate fermentation of the biofilm of plaque, and therefore the rate of caries formation, gingivitis, and periodontitis.

Research confirms this important role of salivary health, thereby adding another dimension to both the diagnosis of overall oral ecology and its treatment. One study found that in children free of caries, 90 percent had normal levels of hydration and salivary flow rate and 100 percent had healthy salivary pH, whereas in the group with caries the rates for these three parameters were all around 30 percent, a significant statistical difference. (6) Similar results have been found in related studies examining other parameters of salivary health, such as levels of calcium and antimicrobial peptides. (7)(8)

It is interesting to note that the sympathetic and parasympathetic nervous systems stimulate production of two different types of saliva. That produced by sympathetic stimulation is thicker and primarily for supporting respiratory functions, while that produced by parasympathetic stimulation is more watery and facilitates digestion. Furthermore, parasympathetic stimulation also increases blood flow to the salivary glands, which in turn stimulates more flow of saliva.

The implication of this is that stress affecting the sympathetic nervous system not only affects digestive health but also weakens and disrupts the ecology of the mouth, leading to an increased propensity for inflammation and infection or a worsening of preexisting conditions. Additionally, many other factors such as diet and smoking cause reduced salivary flow; dryness of the mouth is a common side effect of many prescription drugs.

Gathering the Jade Juice

Knowing that abundant flow of parasympathetic-stimulated saliva is beneficial for oral and dental health, we can understand the value of the qigong exercise called "Gathering the Jade Juice." This exercise is done by circling the tongue around the mouth and over the teeth to stimulate the flow of saliva, which is allowed to accumulate. Once the mouth is full of saliva it is swished around, cleaning the teeth and gums and releasing more saliva. As this continues the taste of the saliva becomes sweeter and the consistency more watery, indicating its parasympathetic origin. The practitioner then visualizes that the saliva is infused with pure silver moonlight that transforms it into a nectar of healing, and then it is swallowed.

I have personally found this exercise not only beneficial for restoring hydration and a sense of wellbeing to the mouth after waking, when fatigued from travel, or dietary excesses, but also very helpful for eliminating simple digestive disturbances.

Oil Rinsing

Ayurveda describes the use of sesame oil as a traditional method for oral hygiene with numerous benefits. Recently, the technique known as "oil pulling" seems to have become somewhat of a craze in the natural health world, with everything from curing receding gums to growing lustrous hair being attributed to it.

The technique is to take about a tablespoon of oil in the mouth, rinse the mouth with it for ten to fifteen minutes, "pulling" it through the teeth and gums, and then spitting it out.

There is no doubt that this method can be beneficial for the mouth, gums and teeth. Sesame oil has known antibacterial properties, and when combined with the increased salivary flow that is created, it becomes more beneficial.

The range of potential benefits beyond the mouth can be understood from the perspective of Ayurvedic "nasya" therapy, which treats problems of the brain, neck, sinuses, mouth and upper back using medicated oils in the nostrils. There is a clear empirical and functional link between chronic infections in the mouth and those in the sinuses and vice versa, so to treat one system will positively affect the other.

There are a number of other oils besides sesame that can be considered for this purpose. Coconut oil is also antimicrobial, and neem oil even more so. While neem oil has a rather disagreeable taste, I see no contraindications for its periodic use in this way, especially when a more powerful antimicrobial effect is needed, as long as it is not being ingested. Other oils that could be considered would be argan, caulophylum, and just about any other species that is widely used in ethnobotanical traditions for topical applications and especially for culinary purposes.

Herbal Ingredients

The major oral and dental conditions such as caries, gingivitis and periodontitis are primarily infectious processes regulated by pH of the bacterial ecology in the mouth; therefore, it is relatively easy to propose a large pharmacopeia of botanical remedies in various forms that would offer great benefits both preventively and curatively. These species can be organized into wide therapeutic categories, the most important being antimicrobials, anti-inflammatories, circulatory stimulants and demulcents; they can then be classified according to the various forms that they can be administered in, as well as following the Ayurvedic system of the three doshas.

Medicinal plants can be used for dental treatments and hygiene as powders for brushing, as decoctions and tinctures for holding in the mouth, rinsing and ingestion, and made into paste for applying as poultices to the gums. Some species can be chewed and used as tooth sticks.

Tooth Sticks

Tooth sticks are small branches, twigs or roots of medicinal trees or shrubs that are used for dental hygiene. A tooth stick is prepared by chewing one end until it is soft and frayed and then using it as a toothbrush and toothpick for cleaning the teeth and gums.

Tooth sticks have several advantages over regular toothbrushes. Where locally available they are either free or cost less, they do not require toothpaste, and are able to freshen the mouth without mouthwashes; additionally, many species play important roles ecologically and economically. Most importantly, these species contain strong medicinal compounds such as essential oils and alkaloids that give them astringent, antiseptic, and antimicrobial powers. The drawback of using tooth sticks is that they must be used knowledgably, as simply vigorously rubbing the teeth with them can cause gum damage.

There are numerous botanical species that are used in different parts of the world. The two most famous are neem (Azadirachta indica) and arak (Salvadora persica), also known as peelu; others that are well known are licorice, cinnamon, tea tree, and sassafras. However, in every culture where ethnobotanical medicine is still practiced there are many species utilized for this purpose; in southern India, for example, species of Acacia, Achyranthes, Ficus and Smilax are used.

Arak

Also known as miswak, this is a tooth stick made from twigs and branches of Salvadora persica. The use of this plant for that purpose has an ancient history, predating Islam. It is mentioned many times in Islamic scriptures, such as the instruction from the Prophet Mohammed to "Make a regular practice of miswak for verily it is the purification for the mouth and a means of the pleasure of the Lord."

Arak has been recommended for dental hygiene by the W.H.O.. The branches of this species are high in natural fluoride and silica, as well as having antiseptic and astringent properties. It has been found that arak has an immediate antibacterial effect on Streptococcus mutans. (9)

Resins

A number of resins have been used traditionally for treatment of dental problems and preservation of the teeth; the three most often mentioned are frankincense, myrrh and mastic. Resins can be chewed, used in brushing powders, made into mouthwashes from tincture, and used as essential oils.

Frankincense

Frankincense gum has been chewed for millennia for its health promoting effects, especially in the mouth. The resin tears typically contain about one percent essential oil content, which is released gradually at biocompatible levels into the mouth and digestive tract.

There are many species of frankincense, and not all of the resins are suitable for chewing. Some, like Boswellia neglecta or B. rivae, have an unpleasant powdery consistency and are often incense and not medicinal grade. The species that are best to use, in descending order, are B. sacra from Oman, B. carterii from Somalia, and B. serrata from India. These come in higher grades of pure and clean resin tears that can be enjoyably chewed for a long time. Besides being beneficial for oral and dental problems, the gradual release of low levels of essential oil can have positive effects on the digestive system, respiratory system and immunity.

Various species of frankincense have been studied extensively for their antimicrobial, anti-inflammatory and anti tumor properties, among others. In a study of the use of B. serrata it was found that "Frankincense application (either extract or powder) can lead to remarkable decrease in inflammatory indices" in plaque-induced gingivitis. (10)

Essential oils of frankincense can be used safely and effectively in mouthwash preparations.

Myrrh

Myrrh is another famous resin that has a long history of use for dental problems. It is significantly more bitter, astringent and antiseptic than frankincense and not agreeable for chewing. Myrrh powder is sometimes found in brushing formulas, and more often in mouthwashes as a tincture. It is often combined with goldenseal when a strong antimicrobial and anti-inflammatory agent is needed, as in acute gingivitis. The essential oil of myrrh should not be used in the mouth.

Mastic

Mastic is the gum resin from a species of pistachio tree. It has been highly regarded since ancient times as an effective cleanser of the mouth, gums and teeth, as well as an important medicine for the stomach and digestive system.

It has recently been recognized as having antimicrobial powers, specifically against Helicobacter pylori. It is somewhat difficult to procure as it comes from only one Greek island, but is an enjoyable chewing resin and an even more enjoyable incense.

A Few Important Dental Herbs

The list of herbs from around the world that research is confirming have potential for dental purposes is extensive. These are only a few of the species that are commonly found in easily available natural dental products, and a few from the Ayurvedic pharmacopeia.

Prickly Ash

Prickly ash bark is commonly found in brushing powders. This species was originally widely used by Native American as a toothache remedy and was adopted by the settlers. It was used traditionally for cleaning and drying wounds.

Echinacea

Application of Echinacea root was a Native American remedy for toothache. It has significant anti-inflammatory and antimicrobial powers.

Goldenseal

Goldenseal is a major herb for treating infection in the gums. It is most effectively used as a mouthwash that is held in the mouth. A close relative that is interchangeable is coptis, goldthread.

Lamiaceae species

A large number of herbs in the Lamiaceae family are utilized for oral and dental conditions, including rosemary, mints, lavender, and sages. These are aromatic species rich in antimicrobial essential oils, which are often utilized in dry form in brushing powders, and as tinctures and essential oils in mouthwashes.

Licorice

Licorice roots are used in Ayurvedic medicine as tooth sticks. The powder, paste and decoction for mouthwash are one of the best for soothing inflamed gums and treating canker sores. It has anti-plaque action, is antibacterial, and has anti-carious effects.

Turmeric

Turmeric is an important anti-inflammatory and antimicrobial herb that has an important place in dental care. Curcumin modulates inflammatory responses. A mouthwash of 0.1% turmeric dilution was found to be equally effective as a 0.2% dilution of chlorhexidine (see below) for anti-plaque, anti-inflammatory and antimicrobial powers. (11)

Amla

Emblica officinalis is regarded highly in Ayurveda as a rejuvenative herb. It can be used as juice, decoction or the powder mixed with water as a mouthwash that is held in the mouth. It is also taken internally for a gradual tonification and strengthening purposes.

Neem

Neem is a well-known tree of tropical and arid regions that provides a number of medicinal preparations from its leaves, bark and seeds. Its twigs and small branches are used as tooth sticks, and its leaves and bark are used in numerous tooth powders and mouthwashes.

Neem based mouthwashes have been found to be "Equally efficacious with fewer side effects as compared to chlorhexidine (see below)…in treating plaque induced gingivitis." (12)

Salts and Minerals

Salt

Salt is an important ingredient in many brushing powders. It has antibacterial properties, and an alkalizing effect. Rinsing frequently with saltwater solutions can be beneficial in treating gingivitis.

Sodium Bicarbonate

Baking soda is also commonly found in brushing powders. It inhibits plaque formation and reduces its acidity, supports remineralization of the enamel, and alkalizes the environment of the mouth.

Pearl Powder

A moderately expensive addition to dental hygiene, brushing with pure pearl powder is a contribution from Chinese medicine. It is regarded as having superb cleansing, polishing and mineralizing effects for the teeth.

Essential Oil Mouthwashes

There are many studies confirming the benefits of herbal and essential oil preparations used for mouthwashes. The major purpose of these is antibacterial, and therefore effective for several common dental and oral problems.

When reviewing research studies related to dental health, two products are frequently mentioned. The first is Listerine, which is frequently the standard used for so-called "essential oil mouthwashes." While it is true that Listerine is an example of an essential oil based mouthwash, it is a better example of how marketing and advertising create problems that are then solved, in this case "chronic halitosis," which drove sales and profits of what was previously sold in the 1800's as a floor cleaner and surgical antiseptic by convincing people that bad breath was the cause of their romantic problems.

The recipe for Listerine is useful from the standpoint of understanding how concentrated and powerful essential oils are: 0.042% menthol, 0.064% thymol, 0.06% methyl salicylate, and 0.092% eucalyptol. The remainder of the recipe is water, various preservatives and flavoring agents, and 20 – 30% ethanol, which has been questioned for its possible contributing role in oral cancers. We can see that the combined total amount of essential oil derived compounds comes to a dilution of 0.25%, which can give us a guideline for making our own recipes using complete oils.

The second product is chlorhexidine, a chemical antiseptic antibacterial. It is toxic in high concentrations but widely used in mouthwashes, skin cleansers, contact lens formulas and as a preservative, even though it is linked to anaphylactic reactions at low doses. It is considered valuable for gingivitis and periodontitis because it tends to last longer in the mouth than other compounds.

Essential oils play an important role in oral and dental care and treatments. Because they are produced by plants primarily for immunological and protective purposes essential oils are by nature highly antimicrobial. There are a large number of studies confirming the antibacterial powers of essential oils against a wide range of pathogens, including MRSA; these results are also found in studies about the use of essential oils for S. mutans and its associated infections. A sampling of conclusions from these studies will suffice to show that these highly concentrated botanical extracts have great potential in preventing and treating oral and dental problems; many of these studies have also found that essential oils work faster and more effectively at lower concentrations than chlorhexidine.

"Cinnamon oil, lemongrass oil, cedarwood oil, clove oil and eucalyptus oil exhibit antibacterial property against S. mutans. The use of these essential oils against S. mutans can be a viable alternative to other antibacterial agents as these are an effective module used in the control of both bacteria and yeasts responsible for oral infections." (13)

"The essential oils from Eucalyptus camaldulensis and Mentha spicata significantly retard biofilm formation and can contribute to the development of novel anticaries treatments." (14)

"In vitro biofilm inhibitory properties were in the order Mentha piperita > Rosemary officinalis > chlorhexidine. In vivo experiments on the antibiofilm properties revealed that all concentrations of the oils were significantly more effective than chlorhexidine. In conclusion, essential oils may be considered as safe agents in the development of novel antibiofilm agents." (15)

"Cinnamon oil produced maximum inhibition zone against Streptococcus mutans as compared to clove oil. This is contrary to the popular belief that clove oil is effective in tooth decay and dental plaque. This study shows the potential of cinnamon oil over clove oil in the treatment of dental caries." (16)

Applications

Essential oils are a valuable addition to mouthwash formulas. The simplest way to use them is simply to put one drop on about a quarter cup of water, rinse and spit out. The longer the dilution is kept in the mouth the more effective it will be. Even the strongest of the essential oils such as oregano and cinnamon can be used this way relatively safely, as long as they are not ingested. Common sense dictates that if an oil feels too strong and potentially irritating to discontinue use or switch to another milder species.

The disadvantage of using an essential oil with water, as above, is that it is not miscible, and can therefore be irritating to the mouth, especially with stronger and more caustic oils as oregano and cinnamon. One way to get around that is to add the drop of oil to sesame oil for rinsing, which will emulsify it. Another way is to add it first to a tincture and then dilute the tincture further in water.

My favorite mild essential oils to be used in the above manner would include frankincense, lavender, and eucalyptus; I would consider the use of stronger oils such as tea tree, cinnamon and oregano only in lower concentrations and for shorter periods of time; besides the potential for irritation of the oral mucosa, strong concentrations of essential oils may have deleterious effects on enamel.

Vata, Pitta and Kapha

The Ayurvedic system of the three humors can offer some basic guidelines to help organize botanical remedies into categories that could increase the likelihood of success and reducing the chances that it could cause an adverse reaction. These are simplistic concepts but I have found that there is merit in considering them before giving blanket prescriptions simply because a remedy has a reputation of working for a particular symptom.

Vata

The most basic presentation would be dental and oral conditions accompanied with dryness of the mouth, decreased salivary flow, and receding gums; chronic periodontitis with looseness of the teeth caused by degeneration of bone and ligaments could be placed in this category. A common sense approach would be to minimize use of ingredients that would have a further drying effect such as tinctures of strongly bitter herbs, salts, baking soda, and essential oils, and to emphasize ingredients with demulcent effects such as licorice, calendula, plantain, aloe juice and marshmallow. Although I have found no mention of it in any research, I suspect that a mucilaginous preparation of comfrey root held in the mouth would have excellent gum regenerating, periodontal tendon strengthening and bone mending powers.

Pitta

The most basic presentation would be conditions characterized by infection and inflammation; classic examples would be gingivitis and canker sores. Treatment would emphasize the bitter cooling herbs such as neem, goldenseal and coptis in tincture, decoction or powder forms, resins as frankincense and especially myrrh, soothing demulcents as licorice, and essential oil mouthwashes with milder cooling oils such as lavender.

Kapha

The most basic presentation would be conditions characterized by a mucogenic appearance such as swollen gums, thick tongue coating and thrush. It would be reasonable to assume that hydrating emollients would be the least effective choice, while salts and mineral powders, bitter herbs in various forms, and essential oil mouthwashes with species such as oregano and cinnamon would be the treatment of choice. Ayurveda would suggest spicy stimulants as clove and cardamom, and astringent tooth sticks such as Acacia catechu.

Early American Dental Herbs

Considering the widespread poverty, poor nutrition and lack of medical care that existed in the U.S. and Europe of the 1700 and 1800's, the status of dental health in the general population was undoubtedly very low. Herbalists of the time were probably faced with frequency and severity of tooth decay, gingivitis, periodontitis and other dental diseases that could be found today in some Third World countries. It is reasonable, therefore, to consider that those herbalists had firsthand experience with what plants worked effectively for these conditions.

As a simple example of what can be found in the classical herbals that were used in the early American colonies, here are a few quotes from the English herbalist Nicholas Culpeper about some important remedies of the time for dental and oral problems. "Fastening" loose teeth appears to have been a primary concern.

"If you will keep your teeth from rotting or aching, wash your mouth continually every morning with juice of lemons, and afterwards rub your teeth either with a sage leaf or else with a little nutmeg powder."

"Myrrh fastens loose teeth."

"The juice of purslane used with oil of roses…is good for sore mouths and gums that are swollen, and to fasten loose teeth."

"Mastic…fastens the teeth and strengthens the gums, being chewed in the mouth." "Being mixed with white wine and the mouth washed with it, it cleanses the gums of corruption and fastens loose teeth."

About strawberry: "Lotions and gargles for sore mouths or ulcers therein…are made with the leaves and roots thereof, which is also good to fasten loose teeth and to heal spongy foul gums."

About decoction of goldenrod: "It also is of especial use in all lotions for sores or ulcers in the mouth…it also helps to fasten the teeth that are loose in the gums."

About elecampane root: "The decoction of the roots in wine or the juice taken therein…gargled in the mouth or the root chewed, fasteneth loose teeth and keeps them from putrefaction."

About celandine: "The juice of decoction of the herb gargled between the teeth that ache eases the pain, and the powder of the dried root laid upon any aching, hollow or loose tooth will cause it to fall out."

"Rosemary flower wine…strengthens the gums and teeth."

The Psychology of Dental Hygiene

Unlike many herbal treatments of common ailments, the use of botanical remedies for dental hygiene is an ongoing process that continues throughout life, not just when there are active symptoms. Therefore, a certain mindset is necessary to implement the long-term use of various products if we are to successfully preserve and protect the teeth and gums from the encroachment of aging and decay.

Some people can approach this endeavor with yogic discipline, but I am not one of them. What I have found works best for me is to be faced every morning and evening with a variety of intriguing powders and liquids to experiment with. I have found that it is more effective to brush with an herbal powder one day, rinse with oil the next, use an essential oil mouthwash the following and a tooth stick the next, than to repeat the same routine for months and lose interest. Therefore, my suggestion for maintaining good dental and oral health is to enjoy a variety of new tastes and sensations, which not only makes it more interesting for the years ahead, but probably also creates a more wide spectrum beneficial effect on the complex ecology of the mouth.

References

(1) Amin, O.M. 2003. On the diagnosis and management of Neuro-cutaneous Syndrome (NCS), a toxicity disorder from dental sealants. Explore! for the Professional 12:21-25.

(2) Minerva Stomatol. 1990 May;39(5):413-29.
[The role of Streptococcus mutans in human caries].

Mosci F, Perito S, Bassa S, Capuano A, Marconi PF.

Università degli Studi di Perugia, Istituto di Clinica Odontoiatrica.

(3) Front Biosci. 2004 May 1;9:1267-77.
Virulence properties of Streptococcus mutans.

Banas JA.
Center for Immunology and Microbial Disease, Albany Medical College,MC-151, 47 New Scotland Avenue, Albany, NY 12208, USA.

(4) Crit Rev Oral Biol Med. 2002;13(2):108-25.
A mixed-bacteria ecological approach to understanding the role of the oral

bacteria in dental caries causation: an alternative to Streptococcus mutans and the specific-plaque hypothesis.

Kleinberg I.
Department of Oral Biology and Pathology, State University of New York, Stony Brook,

(5) J Dent Res. 1994 Mar;73(3):672-81.
Role of micro-organisms in caries etiology. van Houte J.

Forsyth Dental Center, Department of Oral Microbiology, Boston, Massachusetts 02115.

(6) J Indian Soc Pedod Prev Dent. 2012 Jul;30(3):212-7. doi: 10.4103/0970-4388.105013.
Evaluation of non-microbial salivary caries activity parameters and salivary biochemical indicators in predicting dental caries.

Kaur A, Kwatra KS, Kamboj P.
Paediatric and Preventive Dentistry, B.R.S. Dental College and Hospital, Sultan Pur, Panchkula, Haryana, India.

(7) Pediatr Dent. 2002 Nov-Dec;24(6):581-6.
Can salivary composition and high flow rate explain the low caries rate in children with familial dysautonomia?

Mass E, Gadoth N, Harell D, Wolff A.
Department of Pediatric Dentistry, The Maurice and Gabriela Goldschleger School of Dental Medicine Tel Aviv, Israel.

(8) BMC Oral Health. 2006 Jun 15;6 Suppl 1:S13.
Oral antimicrobial peptides and biological control of caries.

Dale BA, Tao R, Kimball JR, Jurevic RJ.
Dept. of Oral Biology, Box 357132, University of Washington, Seattle WA 98195, USA.

(9) J Contemp Dent Pract. 2004 Feb 15;5(1):105-14.
The immediate antimicrobial effect of a toothbrush and miswak on cariogenic bacteria: a clinical study.

(10) The effect of Frankincense in the treatment of moderate plaque-induced gingivitis: a double blinded randomized clinical trial.

Khosravi Samani M, Mahmoodian H, Moghadamnia A, Poorsattar Bejeh Mir A, Chitsazan M.

Department of Periodontology & Implantology, Dental Materials Research Center, Dentistry School, Babol University of Medical Sciences.

(11) J Indian Soc Periodontol. 2012 Jul;16(3):386-91. doi: 10.4103/0972-124X.100917.

Comparative evaluation of 0.1% turmeric mouthwash with 0.2% chlorhexidine gluconate in prevention of plaque and gingivitis: A clinical and microbiological study.

Mali AM, Behal R, Gilda SS.

(12) To evaluate the antigingivitis and antipalque effect of an Azadirachta indica (neem) mouthrinse on plaque induced gingivitis: A double-blind, randomized, controlled trial.

Chatterjee A, Saluja M, Singh N, Kandwal A.
Department of Periodontics, Institute of Dental Sciences, Bareilly, Uttar Pradesh, India.

(13) J Contemp Dent Pract. 2012 Jan 1;13(1):71-4.
Antimicrobial activity of commercially available essential oils against Streptococcus mutans.

Chaudhari LK, Jawale BA, Sharma S, Sharma H, Kumar CD, Kulkarni PA.
Department of Oral Medicine and Radiology, ACPM Dental College, Dhule, Maharashtra, India.

(14) Int J Dent Hyg. 2009 Aug;7(3):196-203. doi: 10.1111/j.1601-5037.2009.00389.x.
The effect of Mentha spicata and Eucalyptus camaldulensis essential oils on dental biofilm.

Rasooli I, Shayegh S, Astaneh S.
Department of Biology, Shahed University, Tehran, Iran.

(15) Phytother Res. 2008 Sep;22(9):1162-7. doi: 10.1002/ptr.2387.
Phytotherapeutic prevention of dental biofilm formation.

Rasooli I, Shayegh S, Taghizadeh M, Astaneh SD.

Department of Biology, Shahed University, Opposite Imam Khomeini's Shrine, Tehran-Qom Highway, Tehran, Iran.

(16) <u>Acta Biomed.</u> 2011 Dec;82(3):197-9.
Comparative study of cinnamon oil and clove oil on some oral microbiota.

<u>Gupta C, Kumari A, Garg AP, Catanzaro R, Marotta F.</u>
Amity Institute for Herbal Research and Studies, Amity University, Noida, India.

VI

Cosmic Chemistry
The Effects of Circadian Rhythms and Ecological Factors On the Production Of Medicinal Plant Compounds

Introduction

This article is presented in two sections.

The first introduces a macrocosmic view of life as seen through traditional Vedic philosophy. Using the language of Ayurveda, this view serves as a starting point to understanding the interrelationships among celestial rhythms of the sun and moon, planetary biospheric cycles, the growth cycles of plants, their metabolism of local environmental elements, the production of therapeutically important compounds within the plants, and how those compounds in turn produce their physiological effects in the human body in ways that reveal the underlying cosmological patterns that created them.

The second section describes how these mechanisms operate as understood by modern agriculture, phytochemistry, plant ecophysiology and other related sciences, and attempts to draw some parallels between the language of Ayurvedic and Chinese medicine and phytochemistry.

1: Vedic Philosophy: Life as the evolution of light into consciousness

Traditional Asian medical philosophy is based on the observation of macro-elements and life force energies within the body, and describes their functions and activities in the language of biospheric physiology. The effects of medicinal plants are therefore described according to their tastes, energetic nature and potencies, which define their resulting physiological actions in qualitative terms such as heating, cooling, drying, moistening, and so on. Therefore, medicinal plants can be described as carriers of the elements and energies present in the biosphere that in turn act on those same elements and energies within the body. Simple examples of this include spices as vehicles of fire element, decongestant essential oils from conifer needles as vehicles of air element, sedative herbs such as valerian root as vehicles of earth element, and so on.

In the view of Vedic philosophy, life is the evolution of light into consciousness. By understanding the cosmology that this refers to, we can perceive holistically the flow of energy from sunlight through the plant kingdom into the human body and its metabolism into the nutrients that support consciousness. In this flow the plants act first as receptacles of influences from the sun and moon, second as evolutionary beings that metabolize environmental elements according to their unique forms of intelligence, third as agents that act upon human physiology, and finally as the nutritional basis for supporting consciousness. While pure consciousness may ultimately transcend dependency on external factors, the functioning of ordinary consciousness in living beings rests upon celestial, botanical, and ecological foundations; it can therefore be said that Creation perceives itself.

The sun is the origin of light, which is the creative and transformative power of the fire element manifest as stellar energy. This energy streams into the atmosphere and in conjunction with the earth's rotation is the basis of circadian rhythms created by day and night, the yearly cycles of the seasons, and the monthly lunar cycles. These cycles are the primary influence on the germination, growth, fruiting, seeding, dying, dormancy and regeneration of plants. The cycles of sun and moon, therefore, control the plant world.

The plants in turn bring their evolutionary intelligence in the form of DNA within their seeds; in Ayurvedic terms this intelligence can be described as a latent and concentrated form of *prana*, life force. If traced back through the lineage of individual plant species, this pranic information arrives most recently from the plant species' closest ancestors, then from earlier and simpler plant forms, then from early microbial life, then from the primordial elements, and finally from the origins of cosmos. If we consider Vedic philosophy again, we learn that the physical universe is the external expression of mahat, "universal mind." In this view, it can be said that the genetic intelligence within plants is a microscopic form of universal intelligence, or micro-mahat.

When the celestial influences of sun and moon act upon the ancient evolutionary pranic intelligence within seeds, the cycles of germination and growth begin. As the plant grows, it metabolizes the four basic elements of its local environment, being earth nutrients, water, fire as photosynthesized sunlight, and air as the plant's respiration; these elements are circulated through the fifth element, the channels of space within the plant.

At this stage we can see that what is now present in each individual plant species is the celestial influences of sun and moon, the ancestral pranic intelligence carried within the plant's lineage, and the environmental elements metabolized by the plant. The multitude of chemical compounds found within each plant are therefore the externalized molecular forms of these underlying levels of botanical intelligence (genetics), life force (metabolism), ecological influences, and celestial energies.

Upon entering any field of organoleptic analysis of plant products, such as wine tasting, coffee and tea tasting, olfactory analysis of fragrances and so on, one discovers a language and terminology based on the elements of the environment.

Chardonnay grapes prefer soils that are rich in chalk, clay and limestone; the metabolism of this earth element by the vines adds a flavor sommeliers describe as "minerality." Master tea tasters in China are reputed to be able to identify the region and sometimes exact farm where a specific cup of tea originated; the unique flavor notes present in the same species of Camelia sinensis from different places are the actual tastes of the environment it came from. In my own experience teaching about essential oils, especially in a more contemplative mode, I have found that a group of students, without being told what the species or origin of an oil is, can often come to a consensus about the environment the plant grew in: altitude, climate, soil, water, and so on.

These examples illustrate that what reaches our senses as quantitative molecular information is also the qualitative presence of the underlying ecospheric elements that have been expressed by the pranic intelligence of each species under the overarching control of celestial circadian rhythms. The implications of this are numerous, but the most fundamental is that through the holistic macro-thinking of traditional medical philosophy we are able to develop an awareness of biological interrelatedness, which is the spiritual foundation of ecological sensitivity.

2. Agriculture, Phytochemistry, and Ecophysiology

Agricultural sciences are well acquainted with the implications of environmental influences on plant species, and an abundance of information on plant physiology is available in many disciplines of study. This knowledge reveals the intrinsic mandalic structures of nature referred to by Ayurvedic thinking, although scientific research is rarely concerned with this dimension. In general, the aim of agricultural research is to find ways to increase crop yields, decrease losses from diseases and pests, and increase certain traits and constituents within species.

These goals are also the aim of genetic modification of plants. In the view of Vedic science, gene splicing can be understood as penetrating ancient microscopic lineages of botanical pranic intelligence with toxic parasitic viral vectors that allow the insertion of other lineages of intelligence. While having the above stated goals, this practice is obviously motivated by interest in ownership of those new lineages.

The biotech industry is moving rapidly to create transgenic medicinal plants, and numerous articles with tantalizing titles such as *"Over-expression of Coptis japonica Norcoclaurine 6-O-Methyltransferase Overcomes the Rate-Limiting Step in Benzylisoquinoline Alkaloid Biosynthesis in Cultured Eschscholzia californica"* and *"Metabolic Engineering of Plant Alkaloid Biosynthesis"* can now be found proliferating online. In the concluding words of one such article "Such metabolically engineered plants should prove useful as breeding materials for obtaining improved medicinal components." Herbalists would be advised to consider the approaching conjunction between an exploding global market for herbal products and declining botanical biodiversity and availability, and the symbiotic relationships among biotech companies, pharmaceutical companies moving into production of nutraceuticals, and the medical profession seeking less toxic medications. (1)

Secondary compounds

An important concept in plant ecophysiology is the production of primary versus secondary metabolic products. All plants produce primary products such as carbohydrates, lipids, proteins, chlorophyll, and nucleic acids; these compounds are involved in the primary metabolic processes of building and maintaining plant cells. These primary products themselves may have nutritive or medicinal effects for humans, but the therapeutic benefits offered by medicinal plants are more typically derived from individual or synergistic combinations of secondary metabolic compounds.

To date, approximately 170,000 plant secondary metabolic compounds are known. (2) While secondary chemicals may not have a role in building or maintaining cells, research is now showing that they serve diverse functions such as immune protection, inter-plant competition, and attractants to pollinators and beneficial symbiots. They are also known to give protection against changes in environmental conditions, such as water and light levels, UV exposure and soil nutrients, and to work at the cellular level as growth regulators, modulators of gene expression and other functions. The development of these secondary metabolites is an evolutionary response to the multitude of stress factors found in a plant's environment, factors that an individual plant must confront while being immobile.

In this regard we could consider that in some cases the therapeutic use of medicinal plants is the application of secondary metabolic compounds with specific botanical functions to support or correct parallel or similar functions within human physiology. A clear example of this is the production of essential oils in aromatic plants for defensive purposes, which are then extracted and utilized for their antimicrobial functions in aromatherapy. Another example is compounds produced for neurotoxin effects against herbivores that are utilized for their neurological benefits in humans, such as St. John's Wort. In other cases a parallel cannot be made; the production of valepotriates within valerian probably does not assist the plant with insomnia.

An important aspect of botanical medicine that distinguishes it from allopathic pharmaceutical medicine is that the therapeutic actions of plants are due to synergies of compounds that act on multiple target sites and physiological functions, rather than single xenobiotic compounds. This diversity of compounds and functions originates in the role of synergistic secondary compounds in plants, which together have a higher level of effectiveness than single compounds. Again, the example of essential oils is relevant, which are composed of hundreds of individual compounds working together to produce immunological protection, with the diversity of compounds increasing the potency of broad-spectrum antimicrobial powers and decreasing the likelihood of microbial resistance. As an example, research confirms that tea tree oil is ten times more effective as an antibacterial agent than isolated terpenen-4-ol, its primary active compound.

Ecophysiology

There are a number of important ecophysiological factors that directly affect the production of secondary metabolic compounds in medicinal plants. When summed up it can be seen that they correlate directly with the cosmological view described earlier. These are:

Diurnal rhythms of sunlight and heat (solar cycles, fire element)

Oscillations of lunar cycles (subtle aspect of fire element and influence over water element)

Germination, growth, flowering and reproductive cycles (micro-mahat and botanical evolutionary pranic intelligence)

Antimicrobial, pesticidal, and allelopathic functions (immunological intelligence)

Water, water stress and dehydration (water element)

Soil nutrients and conditions ((earth element)

These influences are present within and around plants from before their germination until completion of their life cycle, and are active in all parts of all plants. The practical importance of this information for herbalists or manufacturers of phytomedicines is to know optimum growing conditions, harvest times and preparation methods to capture peak levels of therapeutic compounds. The spiritual importance is insight into how biochemical medicine is an expression and manifestation of deeper levels of celestial, biospheric and botanical intelligence and energy. The global significance is that all systems of medicine will be irrelevant if biospheric and botanical integrity and coherence continue to deteriorate.

Environmental Stress and the Production of Secondary Metabolites

Among traditional herbalists there has been the understanding based on empirical evidence that wild-growing plants tend to have stronger medicinal powers than those cultivated domestically. From the standpoint of plant immunity, plants growing in the wild must of necessity be hardier to survive; this higher level of vitality would be expressed as higher concentrations of immunological compounds within the plant, either antimicrobial or allelopathic, which are then utilized for human purposes. It could be said therefore that environmental stress is a primary stimuli that creates hardier plant species, and logically stated that medicines from hardier plants confer their hardiness on those who use them, either medicinally or nutritionally.

Modern agricultural research has confirmed that various forms of stress induce the synthesis of a number of secondary plant compounds. It is known, for example, that culinary herbs such as dill, fennel, parsley, and marjoram grown in the field produce higher levels of aromatic compounds than those grown in greenhouses, due to lower night temperatures; higher levels of these compounds means that the plants not only taste and smell better – revealing the presence of more chi or prana in traditional organoleptic terms - but have higher therapeutic value biochemically. This information is relevant to both the commercial production of medicinal plants, as environmental influences can be regulated to increase active constituents, and to those who wild harvest plants, as it can be a valuable guide to when, where, and what part of plants to harvest for maximum potency.

It is important to note that artificially induced stress is now a topic of interest in medicinal plant research. Like many well-intentioned scientific endeavors that lack a greater vision of planetary ecological health, some of these research projects are of questionable intelligence and wisdom, such as field trials that successfully increase production of specific compounds by stressing the plants with metallic toxins or hormonal stressors. (3)

Solar Influences

Sunlight drives chemical reactions within plants. Sunlight levels are measured in lux or lumens; direct outdoor sunlight is in the range of 32,000 to 100,000 lux. Most plants require 5,000 lux and more, and cannot survive below 800, as there is insufficient energy to drive photosynthetic reactions. (4)

Sunlight has a direct influence on the production of medicinal secondary metabolites in a number of ways: diurnal rhythms, photoperiodicy of growth phases such as budding, flowering and fruiting times, levels of heat and light intensity, latitude, altitude and others.

Production of medicinal compounds following diurnal cycles is the most obvious example of the effect of sunlight on secondary metabolites. Diurnal fluctuations in secondary metabolites with medicinal significance have been reported in modern research for a number of species, including saponins in Phytolacca dodecandra, alkaloids in Papaver somniferum, essential oils in numerous aromatic plants, hypericins in Hypericum perforatum, and others. Ethnobotanical traditions also contain such knowledge and experience about cycles of plant potencies. (5)

Many plants produce peak concentrations of specific compounds at noon during the highest intensity of sunlight. For example, diverse species of Hypericum have been found to produce maximum levels of phenolic compounds at this time of day. However, diurnal fluctuations can be expressed at any time of day, such as peak production of carvacrol in Oreganum onites at ten in the morning. Furthermore, even within the same species peaks of different compounds can occur at different times, as in the peak production of thymol at midnight in the same oregano species.

While some species produce maximum levels of medicinal compounds in the full heat and light of the sun, other species require shade to thrive. For example, both the biomass of leaves and roots of turmeric increase significantly when the plant is grown in partial shade as opposed to full sun, and its curcumin content will also be much higher. (6) Cardamom is also a shade-loving plant that has been grown for centuries as an understory crop in old growth forests of India. Species such as these not only offer their medicinal benefits, but are also perfect examples of economically and ecologically sustainable agroforestry.

Shade-loving understory plants, however, are particularly sensitive to changes in their environments and therefore more susceptible to the effects of temperature increases from global warming than dominant woody species. Panax quiquefolium, for example, had a decrease of over fifty percent in photosynthesis and decrease of over thirty percent in root size when grown under simulated conditions of global warming at temperatures of five degrees C. over normal outside temperatures. (7)

Different stages of growth and development strongly influence production of maximum levels of therapeutic compounds. For example, in Hypericum perforatum the hypericins, hyperforins and flavonoids peak at different stages, making standardization of these compounds difficult. (8)

Budding and flowering phases in particular tend to produce maximum levels of many compounds. Iranian savory (Satureja hortensis), like many aromatic plants, produces maximum levels of essential oil during the flowering stage, which is further increased if the plant undergoes water stress at that time. (9) However, budding and flowering phases may simultaneously increase some compounds and decrease others, as in the case of Origanum vulgare var. hirtum, which increases its content of p-cymene at full flowering while decreasing its y-terpinene.

Flowering is a response to changes in the length of day and night; this photoperiodic reaction is triggered in many angiosperms by sensing changes in the solar cycle with photoreceptor proteins such as phytochrome or cryptochrome. The conjunction of sunlight activating these proteins and the internal circadian clock controlled by melatonin allows plants to perceive changes in the length of day and night, which then triggers budding and flowering. (10)

Diurnal peaks frequently overlap with either the budding, flowering or fruiting phase of growth; Hypericum species, for example, produce maximum levels of phenolic compounds at noon, but in H. hyssopifolium and H. scabrum the peak production occurs during floral budding, at full flowering in H.

pruinatum, and at fresh fruiting in H. nummularioide.

Cases such as these, while being of biochemical interest with numerous practical applications, also reveal the macrocosmic patterns articulated by holistic medicine. In some cases there are very clear elemental correspondences between macro and micro levels, such as the peak production of inflammatory compounds in spicy tasting plants at noon on a summer day in the desert. Conversely, many times these correspondences do not hold true, as in anti-inflammatory compounds from different species growing under the same conditions. What holds true in both cases, however, is that peak production of therapeutic metabolites is the expression of a conjunction between the genetic intelligence of the plant (micro-mahat) as it reaches its full pranic potential, the biospheric cycle of the season that activates that potential, and the daily levels of solar energy that maximizes that potential.

Ramakant Harlalka, an Indian chemist, agronomist and one of my mentors once told me: "It is very important to understand the biorhythms of plants, as the sun and moon are responsible for producing sensory molecules. Jasmine grandiflorum, for example, starts blooming from four a.m. onward, and its maximum fragrance intensity is between thirty minutes before and fifteen minutes after the sun rises. This time is known as 'Brahma Muhurta,' or 'God's favorite time,' and it is a very special period in the life cycles of many flowers."

Lunar Influences

The moon plays a direct but subtle role in the lives of plants, and is closely related to the water element. Various lunar effects on plants have been observed over time by different cultures, which incorporated the knowledge and experiences into ethnobotanical traditions. These effects are more pronounced closer to the equator, as the moon orbits closer to the earth than in higher latitudes.

The most basic and universal observation, now validated by modern research, is that plants draw water inward and upward as the moon waxes, and that the moisture content then decreases as the moon wanes.

References from old literature indicate this was once common knowledge. The Roman writer Plinius (23 – 79 AD) advised farmers to harvest their fruit for market at the full moon as it would be heavier, but harvest it for their own use at the new moon, as it would preserve better. (11)

One universal observation common to diverse locations and cultures is that wood from trees harvested at different times of the moon's cycle has different qualities. Specifically, it was recommended that trees be felled on the new moon in the drier phase; this was an important consideration for the manufacturing of products, as it determined how well the wood aged. A number of recent studies have confirmed these practices, including analysis of wood densities and strength, heat values when burned, and other factors. (12)

The Central American indigenous practice of harvesting palm leaves for roof thatching according to lunar phases was recently tested in a joint research project of several US universities, which discovered a significant difference in calcium, carbon, and cellulose content and therefore durability of the leaves. (12)

Bamboo is traditionally harvested at the new moon rather than full moon, as its water content is lower and therefore less prone to rot and insect attack. A biochemical explanation for this is that the phenols and other compounds of a plant's immune system become diluted as the water content increases, causing the wood harvested during the moister phase of the moon to degrade faster. (11)

Another example of increased water within plants during waxing moons is the vanilla orchid. Vanilla growers know that during the waxing moon the vines are more full of water, which means they should not be trained as they break more easily. (13)

In Sanskrit the word for lunar energy is soma; this word also has connotations of nectar, elixir, milk, and the ambrosia of immortality. The two most basic qualities ascribed to the energy of moonlight are cool and moist. This obviously does not refer to the physical moon, but to the recognized influence of the moon on the water element. The gravitational pull of the moon affects tidal changes on large bodies of water and can affect levels in wells and springs, but it is improbable that it actually pulls water into individual trees or plants such as bamboo or vanilla. What is more probable is that moonlight has some type of vitalizing effect on the growth of plants in the waxing phase, which in turn stimulates water absorption and metabolism.

One study measured the growth of various angiosperms (flowering plants) in the spring. It was of course found that their growth rates are influenced primarily by heat and cold, with warmth stimulating growth and cold slowing it; however, it was also found that some species grow more independently of temperatures during the full moon, indicating a vitalizing effect. (14)

About a dozen species of brown algae such as Dictyota, Fucus, and Sargasso have moon-related reproductive cycles. Both fresh water and marine species of green algae (Chlorophyceae) have similar periodicities in reproduction as well. (14)

Moon-related rhythms in higher plants have been regarded as empirical truth by traditional agrarian cultures, and form the basis of different systems of planting and harvesting cycles. Modern research has confirmed some aspects of this, however, reports are inconsistent, with some species growing faster during full moon, others during new moon, and others in moon-related cycles at other times; the commonality of these observations is cyclical oscillations of growth.

One possible explanation for the variability is that the moon's influence does not wax and wane only with the full and new moons, which is the synodic lunar rhythm of the sun-moon-earth relationship, but also on the tropical rhythm of the earth-moon relationship from the geocentric point of view. (12)

Light intensity as low as 0.1 lux during the night can affect the photoperiodic time measurement in some plants. A full moon can reach 0.3 lux in northern latitudes, and up to 0.9 lux closer to the equator. In some species the presence of moonlight causes earlier onset and increased proliferation of flowers, while in others it inhibits flowering; some species have developed mechanisms of folding their leaves to shield themselves from moonlight, which disturbs their internal photoperiodic cycles. Since the production of medicinal compounds is strongly correlated with budding and flowering phases, it is reasonable to expect that increased or decreased flowering in response to moonlight would be accompanied by increases or decreases in levels of those compounds.

Mr. Harlalka also had this say about the moon: "The dawn of full moon days in particular is a very unique time for the development of sensory molecules in the plant kingdom, as well as a very energetic time for animals. According to Indian philosophy, the moon is responsible for creating sweetness. For this reason, people put sweets and herbal medicines under the full moon to receive a shower of nectar, and then eat them in the morning. Likewise, the formation of sweet-smelling molecules like epi-methyl jasmonate in Jasmine grandiflorum is the highest when the moon is in its full power. Roses also produce their maximum fragrance in the morning, especially on the full moon day of April. These types of flowers are harvested before the redness goes out of the sky at dawn, and taken directly to the processing unit to avoid losing those sweet molecules."

Antimicrobial, allelopathic, and other immune functions (botanical pranic intelligence)

Allelochemicals are secondary metabolites that influence the growth and development of surrounding plants and organisms, both positively and negatively; in general they function to protect the producing plant, by either repelling unwanted plants or attracting beneficial organisms that assist its survival. They do this through a variety of mechanisms, such as targeting photosynthetic functions, nutrient uptake, and enzyme activities. Many important therapeutic compounds from medicinal plants are produced for allelopathic functions, including phenols, flavonoids, terpenoids, carbohydrates, amino acids and alkaloids. Like herbal medicines in general, individual compounds are less effective than synergistic combinations. (15)

Allelochemicals could be described as an aspect of botanical immunity that operates in the terrain that the plant grows in. Like many other secondary metabolites, production of allelochemicals increases when plants are under stress from deficiency of water, sunlight, or other factors; when not under stress these compounds may not be produced, or produced minimally. Likewise, when target plants are stressed they become more susceptible to the effect of allelochemicals. (16)

Allelopathic compounds are one of the reasons that weeds and invasive species can aggressively overtake other plants in ecosystems, through suppressing germination and other mechanisms; in some cases these compounds are the source of the plant's therapeutic benefits. An excellent example is Cyperi rotundus, a major herb in Chinese medicine used for conditions of stagnant chi, especially of the liver. It is somewhat ironic that this herb is one of the primary ingredients in the famous formula "Free and Easy Wanderer" and also one of the most invasive plants in the world. In traditional ethnobotanical medicine, a high percentage of plants used for medicines are classified as invasive weeds; the increased use of such species as sources of medicinal compounds created for allelopathic purposes could be a viable solution for their control.

Translated to therapeutic benefits, some allelopathic functions can also be seen to operate within the terrain of the human body. For example, the essential oil produced within eucalyptus leaves, with eucalyptol (1.8-cineole) as a primary component, gives both antimicrobial protection to the tree as well as allelopathic protection when the leaves fall to the ground by discouraging the growth of other plants that would compete for water and soil nutrients.

The parallel in the human body is that eucalyptus oil has antimicrobial powers that operate both in the atmosphere when diffused as well as in the respiratory system when inhaled, where it acts as a decongestant expectorant to regulate the terrain of mucus membrane immunology by discouraging the colonization of unwanted organisms.

In some cases the functions extend beyond the immune function of the tree and its secondary parallel benefits to humans. Azadirachtin in neem leaves, for example, gives antimicrobial protection to the tree with secondary antimicrobial benefits to humans, allelopathic protection that repels other colonizing plants, and also functions as a highly effective and non toxic pesticide for agricultural uses.

This multitude of molecular functions reveals the profound level of mandalic intelligence that operates within nature. It specifically points to the role of plants as agents that first created the biospheric conditions for higher life forms to emerge, and now offer their evolutionary immunological intelligence to protect those forms of life through broad-spectrum immunological strategies that target a wide range of pathogenic microbes and harmful insects while protecting and promoting beneficial ones. It also points to the vast potential of known and undiscovered applications of medicinal plants, not only in the sphere human health, but also for veterinary medicine, agriculture, industry, and other fields.

It has been found, for example, that intercropping Chinese medicinal plants such as Atractylodes lancea and Euphorbia pekinensis with food crops has strong inhibitory effects on microbial pathogens. (17) Other studies have found that medicinal plants can be intercropped with food crops to treat specific plant diseases, such as using Geranium praterise to control potato scab through the presence of antimicrobial compounds produced within the geranium roots. (18)

Studies such as these indicate that medicinal plants have the potential to regulate microbial communities of the soil effectively. A parallel can be easily drawn between the terrain-regulating effect of herbs in the soil and their terrain-regulating effects in the human body. Politically and ecologically, knowing that medicinal plants have the capacity to control soil microbial pathogens is revolutionary, as high levels of toxic inputs to sterilize soils is one of the basic practices of petrochemical agribusiness.

Earth, Water, and Air

In addition to the celestial influences of sun and moon and the genetic intelligence of micro-mahat operating as each plant's pranic immunity, there are infinite variables of influences from soil, water, and air that create its medicinal compounds. What are the unique ecophysiological characteristics of high altitude plants that cause them to produce higher levels of certain constituents than when grown at lower altitudes? What effects is climate change having on medicinal plants, and how will this alter their therapeutic powers? The study of these biospheric elements within the context of herbal medicine offers the opportunity to gain vast insight into biological interrelatedness, with both medical and spiritual relevance.

Due to lack of space, only a few representative examples will be given.

Modern agricultural research describes the effect of dryness on plants as "water stress." The traditional belief that plants from the wilderness were more potent than domesticated species has applied specifically to aromatic plants. It has been thought that aromatic plants from arid regions that live with chronic water stress have higher potency due to higher concentrations of aromatic compounds in comparison to moister plants with higher ratios of water to essential oils. One example of this is frankincense from the driest regions of the desert, the tears of which were referred to by traditional healers as "drops of concentrated sunlight."

A specific example confirming this in modern research is a study that found that the concentrations of carvacrol production in Iranian savory (Satureja hortensis) increased dramatically when the plants were subjected to high levels of water stress. (9) Carvacrol is a phenol, and one of the most potent antibacterial compounds found within aromatic plants such as savory, thyme, and oregano. These oils are also more dermotoxic and gastric irritant than many, with the presence of phenols as a primary factor; in this particular case it could be said that the increased likelihood of inflammation as a result of higher content of phenols could be described as the elemental expression of increased intensity of dryness and heat environmentally.

An opposite example is the effect of water stress on Artemisia annua, which reduces the production of artemisinin within its leaves. In some cases, water stress does not affect the production of primary medicinal compounds: levels of silymarin in milk thistle seeds remain relatively stable under various levels of water stress. (19) (20)

Soil chemistry plays a direct role in the production of some types of secondary compounds in some species. One example is triterpene saponins, collectively called ginsenosides, which are the major secondary products present in ginseng roots. Different ginseng species have different proportions of ginsenosides in root tissue that in turn give different pharmacological properties. Even within a specific species, levels of particular ginsenosides are affected by various environmental factors, including mineral nutrient supply within the soil. This is probably one of the reasons that wild ginseng is universally acclaimed as being a more powerful tonic than cultivated; the renowned old wild roots can therefore be thought of as carriers of a unique regenerative power derived partly from years of accumulating and concentrating mineral nutrients from wilderness soil. (21)

Conclusion

While the study of phytochemistry is immensely important for both agriculture and medicine, my personal interest in the subject is simply as a contemplation that deepens my awareness of nature's beauty and intelligence. The focus of my work as an herbalist and teacher at this time could be summed up as finding ways to articulate our biological interrelatedness with all beings. Without a collective dawning of direct sensory awareness of elemental interconnectedness, the likelihood of our species having a habitable world to reside in appears to be decreasing rapidly, while the awakening of the sensitivity that awareness brings represents the hope of creating a sustainable spiritual culture.

References

(1) Metabolic engineering of medicinal plants: transgenic Atropa belladonna with an improved alkaloid composition D J Yun, T Hashimoto, and Y Yamada
http://www.pnas.org/content/89/24/11799.abstract

(2) Plant Volatiles: Recent Advances and Future Perspectives; Natalia Dudareva a; Florence Negre a; Dinesh A. Nagegowda a; Irina Orlova; Critical Reviews in Plant Sciences, Volume 25, Issue 5 October 2006 , pages 417 – 440

(3) Stimulation of the yield of coriander (Coriandrum Sativum) by mild abiotic stress under field-like conditions; Kuzel, S. Hruby, M. Cigler, P. Kocourkova, B. Ruzickova, G.
Conference on Medicinal and Aromatic Plants of Southeastern European Countries

(4) http://wiki.answers.com/Q/How_does_sunlight_effect_plant_growth

(5) Bangladesh J. Bot. 36(1): 39-46, 2007 June; Morphogenetic and Diurnal Variation of Total Phenols in Some Hypericum Species From Turkey During Their Phenological Cycles; Ali Kemal Ayan, Oguzhan Yanaar, Cuneyt Cirak, Mahmut Bilgener

(6) Effects of Relative Light Intensity on the Growth, Yield and Curcumin Content of Turmeric (Curcuma longa L.) in Okinawa, Japan(Crop Physiology &

Ecology)
Plant production science; 12(1) pp.29-36 20090100; The Crop Science Society
of Japan; Hossain Mohammad Amzad; Akamine Hikaru; Ishimine Yukio; Teruya
Ryo; Aniya Yoko; Yamawaki Kenji

(7) American Journal of Botany. 2007;94:819-826; Physiology and Biochemistry
Elevated temperatures increase leaf senescence and root secondary metabolite
concentrations in the understory herb Panax quinquefolius (Araliaceae)
Gera M. Jochum4, Kenneth W. Mudge and Richard B. Thomas

(8) Study of dynamic accumulation of secondary metabolites in three subspecies
of Hypericum perforatum; Raffaella Filippinia, Anna Piovana, Anna Borsarinia
and Rosy Caniato; Department of Biology, University of Padua, via U. Bassi 58/B,
I-35131 Padua, Italy

(9) The influence of water stress on plant height, herbal and essential oil yield
and composition in Satureja hortensis L.; Zahra F. Baher 1 *, Mehdi Mirza 1,
Mahlega Ghorbanli 2, Mohamad Bagher Rezaii; Medicinal Plants Department,
Research Institute of Forests and Rangelands.

(10) http://en.wikipedia.org/wiki/Photoperiodism

(11) Cosmic trees and traditional knowledge of lunar rhythms: Potentials for
innovative scientific research and bio-compatible applications.; Ernst Zurcher

(12) Lunar Rhythms In Forestry Traditions – Lunar-Correlated Phenomena In
Tree Biology And Wood Properties; Zürcher E.1; Earth, Moon, and Planets,
Volumes 85-86, 1999 , pp. 463-478(16)

(13) http://www.vanillaexchange.com/moon_effects.htm
The Effects of the Moon on Vanilla Plants

(14) Lunar Influence On Plants
Wolfgang Schad
University Witten/Herdecke, Germany
http://astro-calendar.com/shtml/Research/research_Schad.shtml

(15) Allelopathy: How Plants Suppress Other Plants
James J. Ferguson and Bala Rathinasabapathi
http://edis.ifas.ufl.edu/hs186

(16) Ecophysiological Approach in Allelopathy; Manuel J. Reigosa a; Adela Saacutenchez-Moreiras a; Luis Gonzaacutelez; Critical Reviews in Plant Sciences, Volume 18, Issue 5 September 1999 , pages 577 - 608

(17) Effects of intercropping peanut with medicinal plants on soil microbial community
Xie H, Wang XX, Dai CC, Chen JX, Zhang TL.; Key Laboratory for Biodiversity and Biology Technology of Jiangsu Province, College of Life Science, Nanjing Normal University, Nanjing

(18) Medicinal Plants for Suppressing Soil Borne Plant Diseases: Suppressive Effect of Geranium Pratense L. on Common Scab of Potato and Identification of the Active Compound; Soil science and plant nutrition; 44(2) pp.157-165 19980600; Japanese Society of Soil Science and Plant Nutrition; Ushiki Jun; Tahara Satoshi; Hayakawa Yoshihiko; Tadano Toshiaki

(19) Charles, D.J., J.E. Simon, C.C. Shock, E.B.G. Feibert, and R.M. Smith. 1993. Effect of water stress and post-harvest handling on artemisinin content in the leaves of Artemisia annua L. p. 628-631. In: J. Janick and J.E. Simon (eds.), New crops. Wiley, New York.

(20) ISHS Acta Horticulturae 756: International Symposium on Medicinal and Nutraceutical Plants; The Effect of Water Stress on the Growth, Yield and Flavonolignan Content in Milk Thistle (Silybum marianum); A.R. Belitz, C.E. Sams

(21) Plant Physiol, October 2000, Vol. 124, pp. 507-514; Medicinal Plants and Phytomedicines. Linking Plant Biochemistry and Physiology to Human Health; Donald P. Briskin

VII

The Aromatic Journey of Prana

Traditional medical systems such as Ayurveda and Chinese medicine (TCM) are fundamentally systems of "eco-physiology," which describe the functioning of the human body using terms and concepts derived from observing the elements and energetic patterns of planetary biospheric physiology. If students contemplate these principles deeply, they begin to develop a kind of "macro-thinking" that reveals not just the basic elemental correspondences taught in Ayurvedic and TCM colleges, but vast patterns of interrelationships between living beings and the underlying commonalities of biological functions. When this type of synthetic and integrative thinking is combined with an understanding, even rudimentary, of botany, physiology, and chemistry, a truly holistic vision of life emerges. A holistic vision of life awakens a sense of reverence for the intelligence operating within every aspect of nature, and this awakening in turn is the foundation of spiritual wisdom.

The subject of prana is an excellent contemplation for developing the type of macro-thinking that forms the basis of Ayurvedic philosophy. Functioning both at the universal and at the microscopic level, prana unites all life into a unified field yet functions in specific ways within the anatomy, physiology and consciousness of living beings. Any aspect of life could be the entry point for this contemplation, as we could examine the nature of prana in any field of science or in any path of spiritual study and practice.

For the purpose of this article we will follow the journey of essential oils used in aromatherapy from their origin within aromatic plants until their absorption into the limbic system of the human brain and their subsequent impact on physiological functions and ultimate metabolism into consciousness. The subject of aromatherapy is especially relevant for this contemplation on the nature of prana, as volatile aromatic molecules, distillation, respiration, olfaction, and the effects of fragrance on the central nervous system all share prana as their primary elemental medium.

The journey of prana as an essential oil from aromatic plants into the recesses of our limbic systems and inward to states of consciousness must begin ultimately at the source of the elements that nurture the plants.

"All that exists in the three heavens rests in the control of prana," states the Prashna Upanishad. According to this all-encompassing description, prana is the original creative power of the universe, inherent within both Purusha and Prakruti before its projection and manifestation into all levels and forms of Creation. It is therefore to be found in the fertility of the soil, in the nourishment of the waters, in the luminosity of fire, in the life-sustaining power of air and breath and diffused throughout all space. This is the deepest origin of all the healing powers inherent within medicinal plants: the pancha mahabhutas as the expression of Prakruti's prana, made available to nourish, strengthen, and cure all beings.

The biological process of creating essential oils begins with the assimilation of the environmental pancha mahabhutas into the bodies of plants. Being the original inhabitants of the earth, plants have the capacity to live by directly consuming the elements of the biosphere, while humans, who appeared relatively recently in planetary history, are completely dependent on plants for both the food chain and the atmosphere. In this way, plants might be described as "higher" beings living in a "lower" realm of biological evolution.

Using the example of a sandalwood tree growing in the forest of Tamil Nadu, we can observe how the external elements of the surrounding forest are assimilated by the tree: the earth and water elements in the form of nutrients and liquids in the soil are absorbed by the tree's roots; the process of photosynthesis captures the radiant energy of the sun and transforms it into carbohydrates; the air element is inhaled and exhaled through the leaves; these four elements circulate through the channels of space within the tree. Over time these elements slowly undergo metabolic alchemy within the heartwood and roots, resulting in a clear, slightly viscous liquid with a golden-yellow hue that has a rich and subtle bouquet of soft, sweet and woody aromatic notes.

This process is not unlike the creation of ojas within the human body, where nutrients of food undergo transformation resulting ultimately in a substance that Ayurveda describes as the distilled essence of the solar and lunar influences metabolized by the plants we have consumed, a nectar gathered from the flowers of the dhatu agnis.

What is it that guides this assimilation of the pancha mahabhutas and their metabolism within the tree and leads to the final alchemical result of sandalwood oil?

The Kaushitaki Upanishad says: "From prana indeed all living forms are born and having been born, they remain alive by prana. At the end they merge into prana once more. " It is, therefore, the presence of prana that distinguishes a living body from a dead one, whether it is human, animal, or plant. We can infer from this quote that prana is present within the seed, that it is part of the power of germination, that it supports the development and birth of every organism and that it is the sustaining power that supports the survival of every being. We can also infer that it is the force that is energizing the metabolic transformations taking place inside our sandalwood tree and therefore an inherent ingredient of the oil that gradually appears in its heartwood.

However, prana is not only energy, but also intelligence. How many trillions of events are taking place this moment within the sandalwood tree as it metabolizes the elements of the forest environment into oil? What controls the myriad physiological events that occur every instant in our own bodies? What force pumps the heart, breathes the air, digests the food, regulates the hormones, excretes the wastes, fires the nerves, balances the liver enzymes, gives power to immunity? Furthermore, what control do we actually have over these events? Obviously, the human body, and likewise all living things, possess an innate and profound intelligence that knows how to grow, evolve, sustain and multiply itself, in spite of interferences from the negative habits of individual consciousness. Remembrance of our utter dependency on this intelligence, present within us from the moment of conception until the last exhalation, is a profound spiritual practice, another of Ayurveda's gifts to the world.

As in humans, metabolism in botanical species can be understood in terms of prana. The subdoshas of vata, also referred to as the "five pranas," are regarded as the outer manifestations of prana, or "lower" forms of prana that are directly connected to the gross physiological elements of the body as compared to the more refined levels of prana residing within consciousness. These pranas function within the bodies of plants in ways that parallel their functions in the human body. Prana vata could be described as the plant's metabolic intelligence that governs its respiration, intake of nutrition, and immunological power; udana vata is the plant's exhalation cycle; samana vata is assimilation of nutrients within the plant's tissues and cells; vyana vata is the plant's circulatory power; and apana vata is the plant's excretory system.

While sharing these similarities of pranic functions with humans, plants have one fundamental difference: they do not have nervous systems as the primary conduit for prana. Here we might postulate that plants do not have sthula prana, the prana connected to a physical nervous system, but that they have sukshma prana, the prana that flows through a subtle nervous system, or at least some form of nadis. This hypothesis is plausible if we consider that there are many documented experiments proving that plants have sentient awareness in spite of lacking a physical nervous system, expressed by liking and disliking of different kinds of music, responsiveness to individuals, and so on.

Approximately ten percent of plants produce essential oils. The biological process of creating essential oil molecules within a plant is referred to as a "secondary metabolic pathway," meaning that it occurs subsequent to more fundamental physiological processes.

It is interesting to note that most aromatic plants are not vulnerable to common pathogens and pests that affect non-aromatic plants; it is therefore likely that the appearance of these secondary metabolic pathways represent botanical immunological evolution. What is even more intriguing is the historical evidence that those who have worked with essential oils during times of epidemics, such as distillers, perfumers, and physicians specializing in the use of aromatic medicines, were less vulnerable to contagious illnesses than the general population. This empirical observation points to the possibility that chronic exposure to the aromatic molecules produced by enhanced botanical immunity has the potential to stimulate, enhance, or somehow educate human immunological responses, a possibility that is now receiving increased attention among researchers.

It is also fascinating to discover that after millions of years of gradual evolution during the early formative stages of the biosphere, the sudden appearance of flowers and their aromatic attractant molecules within the botanical realm was the original stimulus for the explosion of biodiversity in our current planetary epoch, culminating in the appearance of Homo sapiens. In other words, we are the descendants of flowers.

Here we can observe more dimensions of prana at work within the world of aromatic plants. The first is the appearance of essential oils as a botanical evolutionary development; likewise, prana is the force behind evolutionary processes, the unfolding of Prakruti through time and space, whether it is evolution within species based on adaptation or spiritual evolution within an individual. The second is the biological role of essential oils in plants as immunity from a wide range of pathogens; likewise, prana is a fundamental aspect of immunological strength and potency. The third is the affinity that volatile aromatic molecules have with the air and space elements that promote the diffusivity of their attractant and repellant molecules into the atmosphere around the plant; likewise, the elemental nature of prana is that of air and space.

A perfect example of prana functioning within these dimensions is a conifer forest. The air and space (prana) of the forest is diffused with the rich, sweet, balsamic green notes of the essential oils produced by the trees. These oils are the expressions of the trees' collective immunological intelligence (prana), which we could call a type of "community immunity." This intelligence developed over time in response to exposure to multitudes of pathogens, and represents evolutionary forces (prana) at work within the trees.

In this example of the conifer forest there are direct anatomical and physiological parallels that point to the deep underlying biological unity between humans and plants. The lungs have a similar anatomical structure to trees: the trachea is the trunk, the bronchi are the large branches, bronchioles are smaller branches, and alveoli are the leaves. Likewise, the majority of essential oils used for treating upper respiratory conditions and mucous membranes of the lungs are derived from the leaves of trees, such as eucalyptus and tea tree, or from needles of conifers such as pine, spruce, and fir. In Chinese medical terms, the antimicrobial, decongestant, mucolytic and immune-enhancing properties of these oils are specifically for treating "wind cold" and "wind heat," i.e. airborne pathogens affecting the upper respiratory system; likewise, the oils produced within the leaves and needles are released by the trees directly into the air to be carried on the wind. Here we find one of prana's most important definitions, given by the ancient Greek physicians and philosophers: "pneuma," the "breath of life," upon which we are directly, inseparably, and biologically dependent with each respiration.

For many people who are familiar with both Ayurveda and Chinese medicine, prana and chi are similar, if not synonymous, concepts. Like prana, chi is a fundamental principle underlying both medicine and spiritual practice. Like prana, it is conceived as a vital energy that is part of every living thing. Like prana, the flow of chi is described as being associated with both respiration and with subtle and refined currents within a non-physical nervous system: the meridians and acupuncture points. Like prana, chi is the foundation of health, vitality, and immunity, while its disturbance and decline are the cause and result of illness. Like prana, chi is also described in macrocosmic terms, such as tian chi, "sky breath," used in ordinary language for "weather."

The Chinese character for chi is comprised of two ideograms that signify "steam rising from rice as it cooks." In medical terminology this image describes the vaporous essence that is released from nutrients under the influence of digestive fire: the pranic energy of food released from rasa under the influence of agni.

This image also offers an excellent analogy for the process of distillation of essential oils.

During distillation, fresh aromatic plant material is placed inside the still, either submerged in water or subjected to steam. As the water boils, the heat breaks apart the cells containing essential oils, releasing the volatile constituents. The aromatic steam, consisting of water and volatile constituents, rises from the still, travels through a condensing coil, and emerges as aromatic water. The volatile molecules then separate, creating a layer of essential oil and a layer of hydrosol.

What exactly is this fragrant liquid that we have extracted from the aromatic plants? Analysis with gas chromatography would reveal that it is composed of a complex mixture of molecules - terpenes, phenols, aldehydes, alcohols, esters, oxides, ketones – each of which can produce a wide range of effects on the doshas and dhatus. If we look deeply into the origin and nature of these molecules with the universal macro-thinking of Ayurveda, we realize that an essential oil is not an inert liquid, a collection of compounds devoid of life, but the distilled essence of prana: the cosmic prana of Prakruti, projected into the earthly pancha mahabhutas, assimilated by the metabolic power of botanical prana and alchemically refined into molecular expressions of pranic immunological intelligence.

The journey of prana has reached the stage where we now hold it in our hands as an essential oil in a bottle. It is now ready to continue to its last phase: to be used in aromatherapy, where it will directly influence the prana of our respiratory, circulatory, neurological, and immunological functions.

Although there are ways to use essential oils orally and topically, the safest and generally most effective way is through olfaction. Ayurveda states, with a valid logic of natural correspondences, that the sense of smell is connected to the earth element, and the element of air relates to the sense of touch; simple observation, on the other hand, would link the sense of smell more directly to air, as that is the primary elemental vehicle that carries diffusive aromatic molecules. Furthermore, aromatic molecules pass through space, not only that between the source of the aroma and the nose, but ultimately the space within the sinus cavities. Now, we can see the affinity between atmospheric air and space, aromatic diffusivity and inhalation into the sinus cavities as one unified field of prana.

As the aromatic molecules pass from the flower, root, spice, or bottle of essential oil into the sinus cavity, we can observe how prana links the inward conscious to the outer world, and how it brings about the inner perception of external phenomena.

Neurologically, meaning governed by prana, all perception of the outer world arises through a three-phase process. The first phase occurs as sensory stimulation to the peripheral nervous system caused by different types of energies: radiant energy of light, chemical energy of taste and smell, thermal energy of heat and cold, mechanical energy of pressure and movement, kinetic energy of sound vibration. All of these energies could be described variously as forms of prana, the forms that act as the expression of prana, the vehicles that carry prana, or a combination of all.

As each of these forms of energy reach the body, they stimulate receptor sites on the nerve endings of the sense organs. In the sense of smell, aromatic molecules bind at the receptor sites of the olfactory nerves, located in the olfactory epithelium in the sinus cavity. In this first phase of perception, external energies are "decoded" as they stimulate the receptor sites and transformed into bioelectrical energy of neuronal stimulation. In other words, the various forms of environmental pranic energies are changed into nerve current, another form of prana. This pranic transformation can be thought of as taking place within the fires of agni, as the various metabolic pathways between receptor site stimulation and neuronal activation occur with corresponding enzymatic processes.

The second phase of perception occurs as the nerve current passes into the central nervous system and the brain. In the case of smell, this means the neurological impulse, prana, passing from the olfactory epithelium into increasingly large branches of the olfactory nerve, across the cribriform plate of the skull and finally into the limbic system at the olfactory bulb.

The third phase occurs as the prana of neurological current spreads across the neural networks in the brain and stimulates the endocrine glands. These synaptic networks could be said to be under the control of prana vata, the subdosha that governs the senses and consciousness, assimilates sensory information, feelings and knowledge, and in turn controls the other subdoshas of pitta and kapha that reside within the brain. As the electromagnetic holographs of prana arise and dissolve within the brain, corresponding sensations arise within the mind, internal recreations mirroring the three-times-removed realities of the outer world.

Simultaneously, as each breath is inhaled, the aromatic molecules of our

essential oil pass into the respiratory system, penetrate through the water element of the mucus membrane of the lungs, and begin their journey through
the circulatory system, once again under the influence of the five pranas gov-
erning physiological activities.

Here the aromatic journey of prana is completed: from the cosmic prana of
Prakruti to Her manifestations within the universal elements; assimilated into
plants by their life force, metabolized into fragrant molecules by their immunological intelligence; released into the atmosphere as botanical "community
immunity" and distilled as a living pranic vapor; inhaled into the space of the
sinus cavities, transformed into holographic neural networks; carried into the
lungs with each breath of life, circulated throughout the body by its pranic
currents, until they are released once again into the atmosphere.

VIII

Fragrance and Consciousness

Introduction

This paper presents a brief overview of current research into the effects of fragrance on consciousness. It specifically examines the benefits of using essential oils for treating neurological degeneration and chemo-sensory disorders, enhancing concentration, memory, and learning, assisting relaxation and reducing anxiety, relieving depression and counteracting stress. Most of these conditions can be generally classified in Chinese medicine as belonging to the category of Shen disturbances, meaning spiritual, emotional, and psychological disorders that are both a result and a cause of neurological stress, toxicity and depletion.

Olfaction

In humans, the olfactory region is an area of about 2.5 square centimeters located in each of the two nasal cavities below and between the eyes, containing approximately fifty million primary sensory receptor cells. The olfactory sense is able to distinguish an almost infinite number of chemical compounds at very low concentrations, and is over 10,000 times more sensitive than the sense of taste. Compared to sight, olfaction is more complex: humans use three classes of photoreceptors in the eyes to span the visible spectrum, but smell relies on hundreds of distinct classes of olfactory receptor neurons. Fragrances stimulate multiple areas and systems of the brain, influence the endocrine system, modulate immunological responses, and affect emotional states through their impact on the limbic system.

Like all our sense perceptions, olfaction is a three step process: chemical energy in the form of aroma molecules bonding at receptor sites in the olfactory epithelium is deconstructed and transformed into neurological energy; nerve currents are transmitted into the deeper structures of the brain; these nerve currents are then reconstructed into an internal holographic neural representation of the original information from the outside world.

The complexities and subtleties of olfaction have been the focus of intensive research for decades, and new discoveries are continually emerging. An excellent history of olfactory research and an in-depth review of current understanding can be found at http://www.leffingwell.com/olfaction.htm. Some of the most important aspects of this information are presented here in their respective sections.

Olfaction in Animals

Understanding the role of olfaction in other creatures helps us understand its primitive roots and how this complex sense relates to cognition and behavior.

The homing ability of pigeons has been thought to be due to the earth's magnetic field or infrasound. Research has confirmed that at least in some species and locations, the ability is based almost entirely on olfactory perception of the environment. (1)

Diving birds, such as petrels, use olfaction both to locate food in the sea and to identify their nesting burrows. (2)

Water turtles perceive odors in their aquatic environment. Outside the mating season, both males and females avoid each other through smelling each other's odors in the water, while during the mating season males are attracted to female scents, and females are attracted to being with other females. (3)

The well-documented courtship behavior of captive lobsters is based on the olfactory functions of the female's antennules. Removal of the antennules results in dramatic behavioral aberrations including unsuccessful couplings and mortalities. (4)

A lizard's olfactory ability to sense the odors of predator snakes is dependent on its body temperature, with perception decreasing as body temperature goes down. (5)

In order to find future hosts, many species of parasitic wasps are attracted to the fragrance of essential oils and volatile compounds released by plants infested with herbivore insects. (6)(7)

For butterflies and other flower-visiting insects, colors and scents are combined attractants. For example, Vanessa indica butterflies are more visually oriented: they prefer floral scents from Taraxacum officinale and Cirsium japonicum, but are more attracted to yellow and blue flowers, even if scentless. (8)

Bees have olfactory memories of floral scents that help them recall navigational and visual memories of nectar sources. (9)

These intriguing subjects are now the focus of intensive research and product development, as controlling, blocking, or altering olfactory functions in animals supposedly has numerous potential benefits. Mosquitoes, for example, survive primarily on floral nectars, but in order to feed her eggs the female must feast on blood, thereby spreading malaria. The ability of the female mosquito to find its meal is based on olfaction, which is the basis for mosquito repellant products. Eradication programs using pesticides have generally worsened the ecological aspects of the problem, while synthetic compounds such as DEET (N,N-diethyl-meta-toluamide), natural alternatives such as essential oils, and new molecular interventions have all failed to provide adequate protective powers against mosquitoes for the majority of people living in malarial areas. There are huge potential profits to be made in developing effective, affordable, and nontoxic mosquito repellant products.

Olfaction and Compatibility

Although humans are not as dependent on the sense of smell for survival and reproduction as other creatures are and as we once were, olfaction still operates and influences our deeper biological functions. A simple example is the synchronization of menstrual cycles when women live together, which is the result of pheromones interacting with the endocrine system via the olfactory and limbic systems.

Another example is sexual attraction based on perceived pleasantness of body odor, which is the basis of the multi-billion dollar perfume and fragrancing industries. It has long been thought, and there is now an increasing amount of supportive evidence, that there is a correlation between mate choice, odor preference, and genetics, both in animals and humans.

The Major Histo-compatibility Complex (MHC) is a diverse group of genes that help the immune system differentiate self from non-self; these genes are also involved in the production of the compounds and reactions that create an individual's body odor. From the genetic perspective, attraction to a mate with a dissimilar MHC decreases the likelihood of interbreeding. Researchers have confirmed that there is indeed a correlation between perceived pleasantness of body odor and genetic constitutions in humans, but only when women smelled the sweat of men; men's olfactory systems apparently do not differentiate the genetic desirability of potential mates, or have lost the ability to do so. (10)

Hyposmia and Chemo-Sensory Disorders

Olfactory dysfunction has a profound impact on the quality of life and creates many challenges to good health. As the sense of taste is predominantly experienced through olfaction, the loss of smell leads to loss of taste, which in turn causes nutritional deficiencies as a result of not enjoying food. Loss of smell also increases vulnerability to poisoning by harmful or spoiled food. There is also increased risk of injury from fires, inhalation of toxins, or exposure to gas leaks. (11)

The function of human olfaction declines with advancing age. MRI studies have confirmed that in elderly subjects the major olfactory structures in the brain are activated by fragrance stimulation, but with a lower volume and intensity than in younger subjects. (12)

Decreased olfactory function (hyposmia) is also found in neurological degeneration, such as some forms of Parkinson's and Alzheimer's diseases; it is also found in a milder form in essential tremor. In Alzheimer's both olfactory recognition and olfactory memory are affected. High rates of hyposmia are also found among oncologic hospice patients. (13)

Olfactory testing is now recognized as a valuable method for diagnosing early or pre-clinical stages of Parkinson's and Alzheimer's, as well as for the differential diagnosis of other forms of movement disorders. (14)(15)

Other olfactory disorders include anosmia, the loss of smell, and parosmia, distortion of the sense of smell or olfactory hallucinations. The causes of these disorders are numerous, but the primary causes include upper respiratory tract infections, trauma, nasal polyps, and chronic rhinosinusitis. Many prescription medications are known to cause these and other chemo-sensory disorders; nasal decongestants and over-the-counter preparations such as intranasal zinc gluconate gel marketed for the common cold are two examples. Occupational exposure to toxic substances such as heavy metals and solvent mixtures is now recognized as a cause of chemo-sensory disorders as well. (16)(17)

The Role of the Olfactory Bulb in Mood, Immunity, and Neurological Degeneration

The limbic system controls emotions, emotional responses, mood, motivation, pain and pleasure sensations, and many hormonal secretions. The olfactory bulb is part of the limbic system; it is located inside the cranium directly above the sinus cavities, and receives nerve transmissions from receptor sites in the olfactory epithelium.

One of the functions of the olfactory bulb is protection of the brain from neurotrophic agents such as viruses and toxic dust which can cause neuro-degenerative diseases; this is done through continual regeneration of cell population both within the olfactory epithelium and the deeper associated olfactory brain structures. (19)

Animal experiments have found that removal of the olfactory bulb causes immuno-depression, including decreased proliferation of lymphocytes in the spleen, inhibition of synthesis of tumor necrosis factor, and decreased macrophage activity. Bulbectomy also causes biochemical, behavioral, and morphological changes that are common with symptoms of Alzheimer's disease and major depression, including endocrine dysfunction, decreased serotonin levels, and neurotransmitter disturbances. (20)(21)

These changes are thought to be attributed to dysfunction within the neuro-anatomical areas of the cortical-hippocampal-amygdala circuit - which are also affected by major depression - rather than loss of olfaction alone, which does not produce corresponding symptoms. (22)

Based on this information, I propose that neuro-degeneration and neuro-toxicity from olfactory exposure to ubiquitous toxic compounds in the environment, including hydrocarbon pollution, synthetic aroma-chemicals, solvents, heavy metals, molds and pesticides play a much larger role in a wide variety of diseases and symptoms than generally recognized. It is plausible that conditions such as Parkinson's, Alzheimer's, and different forms of depression not only manifest as dysfunction within the olfactory bulb and related limbic structures, but are also to some degree the result of chronic toxic burden to those structures as well. If this is the case, then a number of other disorders could also be attributed fully or partially to endogenous and exogenous olfactory and neurological toxicity and degeneration, including hormonal, immunological, behavioral, and cognitive disturbances.

In the specific case of Parkinson's, the hypothesis that neuro-degeneration is the result, rather than the cause, of olfactory damage has received attention, and some researchers have proposed that the initial causative event may start in the rhinencephalon (olfactory brain) prior to manifesting as damage in the basal ganglia. The clinical experience of holistic medicine also supports this hypothesis indirectly, as many symptoms originating within and affecting the olfactory-limbic-endocrine-immune axis are resolved by removing environmental toxins, such as depression caused by chemical sensitivities. Clinical trials and empirical evidence of aromatherapy also support this hypothesis, as many hormonal, immunological, behavioral, and cognitive disturbances are benefited or cured using olfactory administration of essential oils. (23)

The modes of action of essential oils and their constituents are diverse, including immuno-modulating, anti-microbial, endocrine-balancing, detoxifying, anti-depressant, anxiolytic, anti-inflammatory, and tissue-regenerating.

It is likely that through a synergistic combination of functions essential oils support a healthy cell population of the olfactory bulb and epithelium and provide neuro-protective and neuro-regenerative benefits, thereby protecting the brain from neurotrophic toxins and reducing or reversing the progression of neuro-degenerative diseases.

Essential Oils for Olfactory Dysfunctions and Neurological Degeneration

Conditions of neuro-toxicity and neuro-degeneration cause symptoms of dysfunction in olfactory and limbic structures. Conversely, activation of the olfactory and limbic structures using inhalation of essential oil vapors has been found to reduce neuro-toxicity and neuro-degeneration and their symptoms. This is not surprising, as essential oil vapors are first inhaled directly into and then travel through the affected olfactory and neurological structures; in other words, essential oil inhalation is the most direct way to administer pure botanical substances to the central nervous system. By blocking nasal absorption of essential oils with procain, it has been confirmed that their effects are via stimulation of the olfactory system and not via absorption by the lungs. (24)

In my clinical practice I have treated numerous cases of olfactory dysfunction, both as a primary complaint as well as an iatrogenic symptom. I have seen several cases of hyposmia and complete anosmia benefited to various degrees through the long-term repeated inhalation of a variety of pure botanical essential oil vapors. Other than systemic steroids, allopathic medicine has little to offer for most of these conditions. (18)

The therapeutic effects of essential oils in these cases could be attributed to a combination of anti-microbial, decongestant, tissue-regenerating, mucous membrane balancing, and nerve-stimulating functions of the oils. These functions have great potential not only for treating the symptoms of chemo-sensory disorders, but for reaching into the olfactory bulb and related limbic structures to treat conditions of neurological degeneration as well.

One example of the potential of this type of treatment is the use of mellisa (lemon balm) oil for stimulating the brain's acetylcholine receptors. Acetylcholine (ACh) is the primary neurotransmitter involved in brain activity related to cognitive functions, and deficits in ACh levels and activity are among the primary neurological factors in the development of Alzheimer's disease. Mellisa has been found to improve cognitive performance and mood and may therefore be a valuable adjunct in the treatment of Alzheimer's disease. (25)

Besides improving memory and cognitive function, mellisa oil is also well-known as a mild sedative which has been found to be a safe and effective treatment for agitation in people with severe dementia. It also has antioxidant properties that may provide protection against the free radical damage that is believed to be a causative factor in Alzheimer's. (26)

Essential Oils for Concentration, Memory and Learning

Numerous essential oils have a historical and empirical reputation for improving concentration, memory, and learning, which is now being confirmed and clarified by clinical trials. Enhancing these cognitive abilities is a complex and multi-system process utilizing a diverse range of olfactory, psychological and neurological functions including subjective enjoyment of a fragrance, adrenal modulation, enhancement of alertness, stimulation of certain neurological centers with sedation of others, and other variables.

One example of the multi-system benefits of aromatherapy for cognition can be found in the case of the common oils lavender and rosemary. When tested for EEG activity, alertness and mood, lavender oil increases beta waves with corresponding relaxation, less depression, and faster and more accurate computation abilities. Rosemary oil decreases frontal alpha and beta power with corresponding alertness, lowered anxiety and increased relaxation, and faster but not more accurate computation abilities. (27)

As a practitioner who routinely uses a wide range of essential oils for therapeutic, meditative, and cognition-enhancing purposes, I have come to regard aromatherapy as a form of neurological training that utilizes botanical intelligence to enhance human consciousness, vitality, and immunity. In a way, this is no different than refining and improving our sense of taste by eating a healthy diet and exploring the range of herbal flavors, increasing our visual acuity by developing artistic appreciation and visualization skills, enhancing our auditory capacity through learning to play music, or developing our sensitivity to body sensations through yoga and meditation. All of these forms of learning bring long-term enhancement of synaptic connections in their respective neurological centers; in the case of aromatherapy this is within the olfactory cortex and other related structures. (28)

The olfactory sense offers unique and interesting benefits for increasing memory through increased neural networking. Fragrance association, for example, has been found to enhance memorization and recall. It has been found that if an ambient fragrance is present in a room during memorization, the memory of the information is stronger if the same fragrance is present again at a later date. (29)

Empirical and documented evidence such as this corroborates my personal experience and validates my opinion that aromatherapy is an underutilized modality which, if applied at a larger social level such as in public schools, has tremendous potential for addressing the epidemic of cognitive disorders such as ADHD, autism and other learning and behavioral disorders.

The memory-enhancing benefits of aromatherapy can be further increased by using specific fragrances that strengthen concentration, enhance attentional processing, reduce mental tension, and improve productivity. For example, jasmine has marked excitatory effects on vigilance (the ability to sustain attention), while lavender has marked sedative effects which benefit those who are hyperactive and stressed. Mellisa oil produces a significant increase in the speed of mathematical processing with no reduction in accuracy, while increasing calmness and reducing negative moods associated with stress. (30)(31)

Essential Oils for Relaxation and Stress

Difficulties of concentration, memory, and learning are intimately connected to mental stress and physical tension, which in turn are major factors affecting productivity and wellbeing both in schools and in the workplace.

One of the mechanisms through which essential oils reduce stress is modulation of the sympathetic nervous system. Inhalation of rose and patchouli oils causes a forty percent decrease in relative sympathetic activity in normal adult subjects as measured in blood pressure fluctuations and plasma catecholamine levels, while inhalation of only rose oil causes a thirty percent decrease in adrenaline concentration. Inhalation of grapefruit oil fragrance, on the other hand, results in 1.5- to 2.5-fold increase in relative sympathetic activity; grapefruit oil is known empirically in aromatherapy as an oil that enhances mental alertness. (32)

In another study, jasmine and lavender fragrances at lowest perceivable concentrations had sedative effects on autonomic nerve activity and mood, in the form of significantly decreases heart rate and production of calm and vigorous mood states. (33)

Mental fatigue is an acute and chronic problem for those who spend long hours working or studying using computers. Sedative fragrances such as lavender and sandalwood have been found to be beneficial to concentration and mental stability, leading to improvement in productivity. Lavender, orange, and rose simultaneously improve reaction times and increase mental relaxation. Chamomile and jasmine increase mental stimulation, and jasmine, ylang ylang, rose, and peppermint improve productivity and help relieve the perception of the workload. The optimum effects of these fragrances are achieved if the exposure occurs at three minute intervals. (34)(35)

Relaxing fragrances have important therapeutic applications in the stress-filled world of allopathic medicine. When diffused in dental waiting rooms, the ambient scent of orange oil was found to have a significant relaxant effect. Female subjects were especially responsive, who reported lower levels of anxiety, more positive moods, and a higher level of calmness. This and other studies confirm not only the anxiolytic benefits of certain essential oils, but the higher olfactory capacity of women over men. (36)

In 1991 Sloan-Kettering Cancer Center in New York announced that heliotropin, the compound that gives vanilla its sweet scent, was the most relaxing and pleasant of five fragrances tested for the reduction of anxiety during a difficult medical procedure. Further testing revealed that patients exposed to heliotropin while undergoing MRI experienced 63 percent less overall anxiety than those not given a fragrance. As a result, many hospitals now offer a novel variety of "integrative" medicine in the form of aromatherapy to calm the mind while the body is exposed to a powerful electromagnetic field and radio waves. (37)(38)

Studying the motility of over-caffeinated agitated mice is probably an accurate model for understanding the stresses of the modern workplace. Lavender oil, especially the Mont Blanc variety, produces the most soporific effect on both normal and agitated mice, while lavender, sandalwood and neroli oils have the greatest effect decreasing the motility of normal mice. (39)

Neroli (Citrus auranti blossom oil) is commonly used in aromatherapy as an alternative treatment for insomnia, anxiety and epilepsy; its anxiolytic, sedative, and anti-convulsant properties have been confirmed. Paradoxically, in the above study, neroli had stimulating effects on caffeine-agitated rodents, indicating that the oil alone works as a sedative and in conjunction with caffeine works as a stimulant. (40)(41)

Another research method which has interesting parallels in modern society is the "forced swimming test" (FST), which is commonly used to measure the effects of antidepressant drugs. Inhalation of stimulant oils such as ginger, thyme, peppermint, and cypress result in a predictable decrease in the immobility of mice, while inhalation of lavender and hyssop oils increases their immobility, even after injection with caffeine. These studies are receiving more attention in the field of industrial and corporate psychology, which seeks new ways of decreasing immobility and increasing motility of workers. (42)

From the standpoint of mental health and social wellbeing in the modern workplace, it would be beneficial to plant an abundance of roses, lavender, chamomile, mellisa, hyssop, sandalwood and citruses in and around office buildings. It would also be helpful to develop and market a botanical perfume based on the essential oil of angelica root, which has been confirmed as having a wide range of pronounced anxiolytic effects. Of perhaps even more interest and relevance to our culture is the discovery that this oil decreases aggressive behavior and increases social interaction among rodents. "Thus," conclude the scientists conducting this fascinating research, "our findings suggest the potential usefulness of angelica essential oil against various types of anxiety-related disorders and social failure," thereby offering an alternative to addictive and toxic antidepressants such as Paxil, which is marketed to counteract "social shyness syndrome." (43)

For those suffering from immune weakness caused by stress and chronic fatigue, inhalation of labdanum, oak moss, or tuberose fragrance restores immune functions suppressed by glucocorticoid released from the adrenal glands due to stimulation by corticotropin-releasing factor derived from the stress-stimulated hypothalamus. (44)

Essential Oils for Depression

Depression is one of the most common reasons for using complementary and alternative therapies. Aromatherapy is used extensively for depression, indicating empirical benefits, but only a limited number of studies have been performed to determine its efficacy. Clinically, many of the oils mentioned previously in different therapeutic categories (neurological rejuvenation, mental stimulation, relaxation, anxiolytic) are known to have positive effects on different aspects of depression, which frequently manifests with other symptoms such as anxiety. It is often difficult to separate depression from pain, tension, chronic illness, insomnia, and fatigue; likewise, studies have found that essential oils have different levels of effects on different aspects of the condition.

A study on the effect of aromatherapy on pain, depression, and feelings of satisfaction in life of arthritis patients found that receiving massage with lavender, marjoram, eucalyptus, rosemary, and peppermint oils significantly decreased both the pain and the depression levels. (45)

In another study, lavender was found to have beneficial effects on both insomnia and depression in female college students. (46)

Another study found that the fragrance of hiba oil, a species of cypress, was an effective, non-invasive means for the treatment of depression and anxiety in chronic hemodialysis patients. (47)

Conclusion

Essential oils have historical and empirical evidence supporting their use for a wide range of emotional, cognitive, and neurological symptoms described by Chinese medicine as Shen disorders. An increasing number of studies now validate their effectiveness, pointing to important new ways of balancing and regenerating the olfactory-limbic-endocrine-immunological axis and its relationship to consciousness, mood, and stress. There is tremendous potential for essential oils to be utilized in innovative ways for the epidemic of Shen disturbances, not only in complementary, alternative, and integrative medicine, but as a major part of public health programs as well.

References

(1) J Exp Zoolog A Comp Exp Biol. 2004 Dec 1;301(12):961-7. Olfaction and the homing ability of pigeons raised in a tropical area in Brazil. Benvenuti S, Ranvaud R. Dipartimento di Etologia, Ecologia ed Evoluzione, University of Pisa, Via Volta 6, I-56126, Pisa, Italy.

(2) J Exp Biol. 2003 Oct;206(Pt 20):3719-22. Evidence for nest-odour recognition in two species of diving petrel. Bonadonna F, Cunningham GB, Jouventin P, Hesters F, Nevitt GA. Behavioural Ecology Group, Centre d'Ecologie fonctionnelle et Evolutive, CNRS, F-34293 Montpellier Cedex 5, France

(3) J Chem Ecol. 2004 Mar;30(3):519-30. Chemo-orientation using conspecific chemical cues in the stripe-necked terrapin (Mauremys leprosa). Munoz A. Departamento de Ciencias Ambientales, Facultad de Ciencias del Medio Ambiente, Universidad de Castilla-La Mancha, Avda. Carlos III s/n. E-45071 Toledo, Spain.

(4) GENERAL BIOLOGY The Role of Olfaction in Courtship Behavior of the American Lobster Homarus americanus; D. F. Cowan; Boston University Marine Program, Marine Biological Laboratory, Woods Hole, Massachusetts 02543

(5) <u>Physiol Behav.</u> 2004 Oct 15;82(5):913-8. Thermal dependence of chemical assessment of predation risk affects the ability of wall lizards, Podarcis muralis, to avoid unsafe refuges. <u>Amo L, Lopez P, Martin J.</u> Departamento de Ecologia Evolutiva, Museo Nacional de Ciencias Naturales, CSIC, Jose Gutierrez Abascal 2, 28006 Madrid, Spain.

(6) <u>Chem Senses.</u> 2005 Nov;30(9):739-53. Epub 2005 Oct 21. In situ modification of herbivore-induced plant odors: a novel approach to study the attractiveness of volatile organic compounds to parasitic wasps.; <u>D'Alessandro M, Turlings TC.</u>;Laboratory of Evolutionary Entomology, Institute of Zoology, University of Neuchatel, Case Postale 2, CH-2007 Neuchatel, Switzerland.

(7) Insect host location: a volatile situation.; <u>Bruce TJ, Wadhams LJ, Woodcock CM.</u> Rothamsted Research, Harpenden, Hertfordshire, UK AL5 2JQ.

(8) <u>Oecologia.</u> 2005 Feb;142(4):588-96. Epub 2004 Nov 20.Priority of color over scent during flower visitation by adult Vanessa indica butterflies.; <u>Omura H, Honda K.</u>; Division of Environmental Sciences, Faculty of Integrated Arts and Sciences, Hiroshima University, 1-7-1 Kagamiyama, Higashihiroshima, Hiroshima, 739-8521, Japan.

(9) Floral scents induce recall of navigational and visual memories in honeybees. <u>Reinhard J, Srinivasan MV, Guez D, Zhang SW.</u>; Research School of Biological Sciences, Visual Sciences, The Australian National University, PO Box 475, Canberra, ACT 2601, Australia.

(10) New evidence that the MHC influences odor perception in humans: a study with 58 Southern Brazilian students.; <u>Santos PS, Schinemann JA, Gabardo J, Bicalho Mda G.</u> LIGH-Laboratorio de Imunogenetica e Histocompatibilidade, Departamento de Genetica, Centro Politecnico da Universidade Federal do Parana, Jardim das Americas, Caixa Postal 19071, CEP: 81.530-990 Curitiba, Parana, Brazil.

(11) <u>Int Arch Occup Environ Health.</u> 2006 May;79(4):322-31. Epub 2006 Jan 25. Olfactory toxicity: long-term effects of occupational exposures.; <u>Gobba F.</u> Chair of Occupational Medicine, Department of Public Health Sciences, University of Modena and Reggio Emilia, Via Campi 287, 41100, Modena, MO, Italy

(12) Functional magnetic resonance imaging study of human olfaction and

normal aging. Wang J, Eslinger PJ, Smith MB, Yang QX. Center for Nuclear Magnetic Resonance Research, Department of Radiology, The Pennsylvania State University College of Medicine, Hershey, PA 17033, USA.

(13) J Palliat Med. 2006 Feb;9(1):57-60. Olfactory function in oncologic hospice patients. Yakirevitch A, Bercovici M, Migirov L, Adunsky A, Pfeffer MR, Kronenberg J, Talmi YP. Department of Otolaryngology-Head and Neck Surgery, The Chaim Sheba Medical Center, Tel-Hashomer, Israel.

(14) Differences in olfactory and visual memory in patients with pathologically confirmed Alzheimer's disease and the Lewy body variant of Alzheimer's disease; Gilbert PE, Barr PJ, Murphy C. Department of Head and Neck Surgery, University of California San Diego, San Diego, California, USA.

(15) Olfaction and Parkinson's syndromes: its role in differential diagnosis; Katzenschlager R, Lees AJ.; The National Hospital for Neurology and Neurosurgery, Queen Square, London, UK.

(16) Laryngoscope. 2006 Feb;116(2):217-20; Intranasal zinc and anosmia: the zinc-induced anosmia syndrome.; Alexander TH, Davidson TM. Department of Surgery, Head and Neck Surgery and Continuing Medical Education, University of California, San Diego School of Medicine, VA San Diego Healthcare System, San Diego, CA 92103, USA.

(17) Curr Opin Otolaryngol Head Neck Surg. 2006 Feb;14(1):23-8. An updated review of clinical olfaction. Holbrook EH, Leopold DA. Department of Otolaryngology, Massachusetts Eye and Ear Infirmary, 243 Charles Street, Boston, Massachusetts 02114, USA.

(18) Curr Opin Otolaryngol Head Neck Surg. 2006 Feb;14(1):23-8. An updated review of clinical olfaction. Holbrook EH, Leopold DA. Department of Otolaryngology, Massachusetts Eye and Ear Infirmary, 243 Charles Street, Boston, Massachusetts 02114, USA.

(19) Neurogenesis in the mature olfactory bulb and it's possible functional destination Loseva EV, Karnup SV.

(20) Immunodepressed status of mice after bulbectomy; Novoselova EG, Bobkova NV, Glushkova OV, Sinotova OA, Ogai VG, Medvinskaia NI, Samokhin AN.

(21) Permanent deficits in serotonergic functioning of olfactory bulbecto-mized rats: an in vivo microdialysis study.;van der Stelt HM, Breuer ME, Olivier B, Westenberg HG.; Rudolf Magnus Institute of Neuroscience, Department of Psychiatry, University Medical Center Utrecht, The Netherlands.

(22) The olfactory bulbectomised rat as a model of depression; Song C, Leonard BE. Department of Biomedical Science, AVC, University of Prince Edward Island and National Institute of Nutrisciences and Health, Charlottetown, Canada.

(23) Q J Med 1999; 92: 473-480; Is Parkinson's disease a primary olfactory disorder?
C.H. Hawkes, B.C. Shephard1 and S.E. Daniel2

(24) Recovery of PFC in mice exposed to high pressure stress by olfactory stimulation with fragrance. Shibata H, Fujiwara R, Iwamoto M, Matsuoka H, Yokoyama M M International Journal of Neuroscience

(25) Modulation of mood and cognitive performance following acute administration of single doses of Melissa officinalis (Lemon balm) with human CNS nicotinic and muscarinic receptor-binding properties.

(26) Aromatherapy as a safe and effective treatment for the management of agitation in severe dementia: the results of a double-blind, placebo-controlled trial with Melissa.; Ballard CG, O'Brien JT, Reichelt K, Perry EK. Wolfson Research Centre, Newcastle General Hospital, Institute for Ageing and Health, Newcastle upon Tyne, United Kingdom.

(27) Aromatherapy positively affects mood, EEG patterns of alertness and math computations. Diego MA, Jones NA, Field T, Hernandez-Reif M, Schanberg S, Kuhn C, McAdam V, Galamaga R, Galamaga M. University of Miami School of Medicine, USA.

(28) Learning-induced long-term synaptic modifications in the olfactory cortex.; Brosh I, Barkai E. Center for Brain and Behavior, Faculty of Sciences, University of Haifa, Haifa 31905, Israel.

(29) Verbal memory elicited by ambient odor; Smith D G, Standing L, De Man A; Perceptual & Motor Skills

(30) Effects of essential oils on human attentional processes. Ilmberger I,

Rupp J, Karamat C, Buchbauer G Programme Abstracts - 24th International Symposium on Essential Oils

(31) Attenuation of laboratory-induced stress in humans after acute administration of Melissa officinalis; Kennedy DO, Little W, Scholey AB. Human Cognitive Neuroscience Unit, Division of Psychology, University of Northumbria

(32) Effects of fragrance inhalation on sympathetic activity in normal adults. Haze S, Sakai K, Gozu Y. Product Development Center, Shiseido Co., Ltd., Hayabuchi, Yokohama, Japan

(33) Eur J Appl Physiol. 2005 Oct;95(2-3):107-14. Epub 2005 Jun 23.Sedative effects of the jasmine tea odor and (R)-(-)-linalool, one of its major odor components, on autonomic nerve activity and mood states. Kuroda K, Inoue N, Ito Y, Kubota K, Sugimoto A, Kakuda T, Fushiki T. Laboratory of Nutrition Chemistry, Division of Food Science and Biotechnology, Graduate School of Agriculture, Kyoto University, Kitashirakawa Oiwake-cho, Japan.

(34) A study of fragrance on working environment characteristics in VDT work activities. Kawakami M, Aoki S, Ohkubo T; International Journal of Production Economics

(35) Psychophysiological studies of fragrance; Sugano H, Sato N; Chemical Senses

(36) Physiol Behav. 2000 Oct 1-15;71(1-2):83-6. Ambient odor of orange in a dental office reduces anxiety and improves mood in female patients. Lehrner J, Eckersberger C, Walla P, Potsch G, Deecke L. Neurological Clinic, University of Vienna, Vienna, Austria.

(37) http://www.vanilla.com/html/leg-calmdown.html

(38) http://www.shepherd.org/shepherdhomepage.nsf/0/023e-33c787746713852569a400765211?OpenDocument

(39) Fragrance compounds and essential oils with sedative effects upon inhalation. Buchbauer G, Jirovetz L, Jager W, Plank C, Dietrich H Journal of Pharmaceutical Sciences

(40) Evidence of the sedative effects of neroli oil, citronellal and phenylethyl acetate on mice. Jager W, Buchbauer G, Jirovetz L, Dietrich H, Plank C

Journal of Essential Oil Research

(41) Biol Pharm Bull. 2002 Dec;25(12):1629-33. Anxiolytic and sedative effects of extracts and essential oil from Citrus aurantium L. Carvalho-Freitas MI, Costa M. Department of Pharmacology, Institute of Bioscience, Sao Paulo State University (UNESP), Botocatu, Brazil.

(42) Arch Pharm Res. 2005 Jul;28(7):770-4. Stimulative and sedative effects of essential oils upon inhalation in mice. Lim WC, Seo JM, Lee CI, Pyo HB, Lee BC. R&D Center, Hanbul Cosmetics Co. Ltd., 72-7 Yongsung-ri, Samsung-Myun, Chungbuk 369-830, Korea.

(43) Pharmacol Biochem Behav. 2005 Aug;81(4):838-42. The effects of angelica essential oil in social interaction and hole-board tests. Min L, Chen SW, Li WJ, Wang R, Li YL, Wang WJ, Mi XJ. Department of Pharmacology, Shenyang Pharmaceutical University, Box 41, 103 Wenhua Road, 110016 Shenyang, PR China.

(44) Recovery of PFC in mice exposed to high pressure stress by olfactory stimulation with fragrance. Shibata H, Fujiwara R, Iwamoto M, Matsuoka H, Yokoyama M M International Journal of Neuroscience

(45) Taehan Kanho Hakhoe Chi. 2005 Feb;35(1):186-94. The effects of aromatherapy on pain, depression, and life satisfaction of arthritis patients Kim MJ, Nam ES, Paik SI. College of Nursing, The Catholic University of Korea, Korea.

(46) Taehan Kanho Hakhoe Chi. 2006 Feb;36(1):136-43. Effects of lavender aromatherapy on insomnia and depression in women college students. Lee IS, Lee GJ. Department of Nursing, Keukdong College, Korea.

(47) Psychological effects of aromatherapy on chronic hemodialysis patients Authors: Itai T.; Amayasu H.; Kuribayashi M.; Kawamura N.; Okada M.; Momose A.; Tateyama T.; Narumi K.; Uematsu W.; Kaneko S. Source: Psychiatry and Clinical Neurosciences, Volume 54, Number 4, August 2000, pp.

IX

The Anti-Microbial Effects of Essential Oils

History

Essential oil-containing aromatic plants have been used for anti-infectious purposes for millennia. Sewage, rotting garbage, sick people, environmental pollution, and other sources of unpleasant smells reveal the presence of proliferating microbial toxins. Without knowing the details of what pathogenic agents were present, people understood that where there were bad vapors, diseases lurked. Aromatic plants have been the primary antidote for these 'evil spirits.' Traditional medical systems, such as Ayurveda, had a general concept of microscopic pathogens and knew that substances such as essential oils counteracted those toxins.

Historically, people have known that essential oils had many uses, including medicines and preservatives of foods. The medicinal powers of essential oils have been utilized in various forms for millennia, such as unguents, lotions, perfumes, perfumed waters, fragrant baths and massage, incense, and innumerable other preparations. Essential oil preparations were highly esteemed by the ancient physicians. Essential oil-containing spices were one of the primary methods of food preservation; the search for those spices led to the discovery of the New World.

The anti-microbial actions of essential oils are one of the most extensively studied aspects of botanical medicine. Research into the antiseptic properties of essential oils has been going on since the 1880's, starting with oils such as oregano, cinnamon, and clove. By the 1930's a considerable amount of conclusive studies had been amassed, including proof that essential oils used in perfumes had antibiotic powers, but these were eclipsed by the discovery of penicillin and the emergence of antibiotic drugs. The origins of the current aromatherapy movement can be credited largely to the research and work of people such as Dr. Jean Valnet in the 1960's.

Essential Oil Research

Thousands of studies on the anti-microbial effects of essential oils are available online in hundreds of databases and journals. Research has been conducted on a vast array of essential oils and essential oil constituents from a multitude of species, varieties and chemotypes of aromatic plants, including details of their geographic origins, harvesting and extraction, analytical methods, and comparative results.

Many of these studies have been performed on aromatic plants with a known history of use in ethnobotanical medicine. In these cases, testing the plant's oil components against microbial strains frequently confirms what local practitioners have known. In some cases new information emerges which might improve the use of the plant. For example, the entire aerial portion of a species may be used traditionally for anti-infectious purposes, but testing will reveal that the strongest concentrations of effective compounds are in the leaves rather than the flowers, or that the flowers contain properties that are best used in other ways.

Frequently, the oils used in research are distilled in small quantities for the purpose of the study only, and are therefore not found on the market. Bringing these oils into commerce would expand the range of natural medicines available to practitioners, create new products, and give farmers new sources of income.

The body of research includes not only examination of the antibiotic, antiviral, and anti-fungal properties of the oils, but other important functions including anti-inflammatory, immune-stimulating, hormone-regulating, anti-parasitic, and anti-cancer powers. Furthermore, the research is not limited to human health and medical applications, but extends to other important fields including veterinary medicine, food preservation, natural flavoring and fragrancing, industrial applications, and agricultural uses such as pesticides and fertilizers.

Even a brief perusal of the available literature reveals that essential oils represent a vast and underutilized botanical resource, a non-toxic and ecologically sustainable industry capable of replacing a high percentage of the toxic fossil fuel-derived chemical compounds now routinely used in almost every consumer product. Essential oils are steadily moving to the next level of practical application in a new generation of non-toxic products; this will reduce the toxic biological burden at the root of countless diseases and hasten the transition from unsustainable fossil fuel-based economies and industries to sustainable plant-based economies and industries. This is the true potential of botanical medicines: agents of healing on all levels, including ecological, agricultural, industrial, economic, and medical.

In the field of natural medicine, essential oils are important anti-infectious and anti-microbial agents, whose importance grows as microbial resistance to antibiotic and antiviral drugs increases. Research papers frequently conclude with the observation that these oils are promising alternatives for standard anti-microbial drugs. The challenge in applying this information is making the transition from in-vitro studies on pure microbial strains grown in petri dishes to the realities of human physiology.

Because of their potency and documented pharmaceutical efficacy, essential oils represent an important interface between allopathic and herbal systems of medicine; as their antibiotic powers are recognized they will first replace routine prescriptions for easily treatable conditions, and will later be applied to more serious conditions.

Testing Oils for Antimicrobial Properties

Essential oils are being tested in-vitro, in-vivo in animals, and in human clinical trials.

In-vitro testing of essential oils against microbial strains generally proceeds in three stages. The first step is distillation of the oil from a specific species of plant. The second is analysis of the chemical constituents of the oil, done through gas chromatography. The third is in-vitro testing of the oil or its primary compounds against various strains of microbes.

The most commonly used in-vitro method for determining which pathogens are susceptible to which oils or oil constituent is the agar diffusion technique; this is the same method used to determine the bactericidal activity of antibiotic drugs. The procedure begins by inoculating a standardized microbial strain on agar medium. A series of sterile paper disks are saturated with different oils at different concentrations, and placed over the culture; alternately, the oil is dropped directly into holes in the medium. After a latency period the inhibition halo around the disks is measured, and the anti-microbial activity of the oil is rated according to its size and essential oil concentration.

Although the agar diffusion technique is the most commonly used, it is not necessarily the most accurate, as the essential oils have volatile as well as aqueous properties. Newer methods are now being employed to test the anti-microbial effects of essential oil vapors, rather than direct aqueous contact on disks. Results show that the concentrations of oils needed in the vapor state are far less than when applied in agar medium, thus confirming that not only are the oils highly anti-microbial, but that they are also more potent than originally thought.

The Role of Essential Oil Production in Plant Physiology

Traditional medical systems such as Ayurveda and Chinese medicine are fundamentally systems of "eco-physiology," which describe the functioning of the human body using terms and concepts derived from observing the elements and energetic patterns of planetary biospheric physiology. If students contemplate these principles deeply, they begin to develop a kind of "macro-thinking" that reveals not just the basic elemental correspondences taught in acupuncture colleges, but vast patterns of interrelationships between living beings and the underlying commonalities of biological functions. When this type of synthetic and integrative thinking is combined with an understanding, even rudimentary, of botany, physiology, and chemistry, a truly holistic vision of life emerges. A holistic vision of life awakens a sense of reverence for the intelligence operating within every aspect of nature, and this awakening in turn is the foundation of spiritual wisdom.

In the field of essential oil chemistry, numerous parallels and examples of biological unity can be discovered using this macro-thinking at the intuitive level, which reveal why and how essential oils work. The lungs, for example, have a similar structure to trees: the trachea is the trunk, the bronchi are the large branches, bronchioles are smaller branches, and alveoli are the leaves. Likewise, the majority of essential oils used for treating upper respiratory conditions and the mucous membrane level of the lungs are derived from the leaves of trees, such as eucalyptus and ravensare, or from needles of conifers such as pine, spruce, and fir. In Chinese medical terms, these oils are specifically for Wind Cold and Wind Heat, i.e. airborne pathogens; likewise, the oils produced within these leaves and needles are released directly into the air.

The immunological functions of essential oils within plants are also directly related to their effects on human immunity. Essential oils are secondary metabolic byproducts which serve several physiological purposes, including anti-bacterial, anti-vital, and wound healing. The molecules within an essential oil can be thought of as the expression of the plant's immunological intelligence; when we utilize essential oils we are using botanical immuno-chemical intelligence to repel and destroy pathogens common to both plants and humans, and to activate healing processes that are likewise similar in both. It is interesting to note that most aromatic plants are not vulnerable to common pathogens and pests that affect non-aromatic plants; likewise, those who have worked with essential oils during times of epidemics, such as distillers and professional perfumers, have a historical reputation of being less vulnerable to contagious illnesses.

Modes of Antimicrobial Actions

Different molecular compounds work differently against different microbes. One of the major models of anti-microbial action that has been confirmed is cellular membrane toxicity caused by monoterpenoid components.

Although essential oils are complex mixtures, research suggests that the monoterpenes, being lipophilic, diffuse into cell membranes and cause them to expand, thereby increasing their fluidity, disordering membrane structures, and inhibiting membrane-embedded enzymes. Studies on the effects of essential oils such as oregano, ravensare, and tea tree show that they cause rapid cellular damage to bacteria. By inhibiting the enzymes and cofactors involved in the respiratory electron transport chain spanning the cytoplasmic membranes of bacteria and mitochondrial membranes of yeast, the monoterpenes cause inhibition of respiratory oxygen of microbes. Even slight changes to the structural integrity of cell membranes can detrimentally affect cellular metabolism. In the case of monoterpene toxicity, potassium ions are lost, which disrupts ionic homeostasis and disturbs chemiosmotic control of energy-dependent processes such as metabolism and motility.

Antibiotic drugs interrupt specific metabolic pathways, such as the formation of a particular protein used to build a cell membrane; bacteria can learn how to resist this specific disrupting influence within ten days of being exposed to the drug. The biochemical action of essential oils prevents this from happening; by blocking the entire cellular respiratory function, bacteria are simply suffocated. Some of the strongest anti-microbial compounds, such as the phenols thymol and carvacrol, can completely block oxygen intake in cell membranes.

Essential oils not only neutralize pathogenic germs, but also help to restore and correct the underlying humoral terrain, such as expectoration from congested mucous membranes, as well as enhancing and stimulating the immune system. Used properly, essential oils do not harm or disrupt beneficial intestinal flora. They are effective against bacteria, viruses, parasites, fungus, and yeast. Because of their wide-spectrum action against pathogens and immune enhancing functions, essential oils are an increasingly important alternative to antibiotic therapy.

Antimicrobial Compounds in Essential Oils

For safe and effective therapeutic use of essential oils it is important to have a basic knowledge of their constituents. Essential oils usually contain several major compounds and many more minor compounds, sometimes numbering hundreds. Researchers have identified many specific compounds responsible for the anti-microbial powers of oils; however, like other herbal preparations and phyto-medicines, the effect of synergies is probably more biocompatible and therapeutically balanced than using an isolated active ingredient.

The chemical compounds in essential oils fall into two primary groups: hydrocarbons, which are mainly terpenes (monoterpenes, diterpenes, and sesquiterpenes), and oxygenated compounds which are phenols, terpene alcohols, esters, ethers, aldehydes, ketones, and oxides. While some compounds are distinctly more anti-microbial than others, there are many adjunctive uses for the less potent anti-microbial oils.

Terpenes

Terpenes, which include monoterpenes, sequiterpenes, and diterpenes, comprise a large group of molecules found in some form in almost all essential oils, with a wide range of therapeutic functions.

Different monoterpenes have anti-inflammatory, antiseptic, antiviral and antibacterial properties; some are stimulating with a tonic effect; others are expectorant and mucous membrane stimulants and decongestants; others are atmospheric antiseptic agents. Limonene, found in most citrus oils, has expectorant and antiviral actions. Pinene, found in pine, cypress, and tea tree oils and cymene, found in thyme oil, have powerful antiseptic actions. Other monoterpenes include camphene (firs, lemongrass, sweet fennel, nutmeg, cypress, valerian); sabinene (juniper berry, cedarwood, rose geranium); and cadinine (hyssop, myrrh, tea tree).

Sesquiterpenes have outstanding anti-inflammatory properties which can be used in conjunction with stronger anti-microbials or for chronic inflammation following infections. The sequiterpene group contains chamazulene (chamomiles, blue yarrow), farnesol (chamomiles, rose), valeranon (valerian), and santalol (sandalwood). Jatamansi (Himalayan spikenard) is nearly one hundred percent sesquiterpenes.

Diterpenes are rarely found in essential oils, as they are less volatile and distill only in minute amounts.

Terpene Alcohols

Terpene alcohols as a group are among the most beneficial and versatile of the essential oil compounds. They have broad spectrum anti-infectious, antibacterial, antifungal, and antiviral properties; they also possess uplifting and energizing stimulant and tonic properties. In general they are nontoxic, non-irritating, and relatively safe.

Two of the more common terpenic alcohols found in anti-microbial oils are terpinen-4-ol in Melaleuca alternifolia (tea tree) and Origanum majorana (sweet marjoram), and alpha terpineol, found in Ravensara aromatica (ravensare) and Eucalyptus radiata. Other important terpenic alcohols with anti-microbial actions are linalool, found in Coriandrum sativum (coriander), thyme (linalool chemo-type), and different species of lavender; geraniol, found in Cymbopogon martinii (palmarosa) and thyme (geraniol chemo-type); thujanol, found in thyme (thujanol chemo-type) and Origanum majorana (sweet marjoram); and menthol, found in Mentha piperita (peppermint) and Mentha arvensis (field mint).

Phenols

Phenols are among the most potent of the anti-microbial compounds. Phenols have powerful broad spectrum anti-infectious and antibacterial functions, are antiseptic and disinfectant, and have strong anti-parasitic properties. They have moderately strong tonic, stimulant, anti-viral, anti-fungal, and immune enhancing properties.

Although they have excellent antiseptic properties, phenols are skin and mucous membrane irritants which can be caustic, especially when used neat. Oils high in phenols should be used in low concentrations and for short periods of time, after which they should be replaced by others that are less potentially toxic.

Three of the most important phenols from essential oils are thymol, carvacrol, and eugenol. Thymol is found in high concentration in oils such as Thymus vulgaris (thyme) and Trachyspermum ammi (ajowan). Carvacrol is found in oils such as Origanum compactum (oregano), Origanum heracleoticum (Greek oregano), Corydothymus capitatus (Spanish oregano), Satureja montana (savory), and Thymus serpyllum (wild thyme). Eugenol is found in oils such as Eugenia caryophyllus (clove), Cinnamomum verum (Ceylon cinnamon leaf), and Ocimum gratissimum (basil eugenol chemo-type).

Aldehydes

Monoterpene aldehydes are found primarily in the lemon-scented oils. This group contains oils that have anti-inflammatory, anti-infectious, anti-fungal, anti-bacterial, and disinfectant powers. These oils must be used with caution as they can cause skin irritation.

Monoterpene aldehydes include citral (bergamot, lemon, lime, lemongrass, melissa), geranial (petitgrain, orange, lemon, mellisa), neral (verbena, lemongrass, lemon), and citronellal (citronella, grapefruit, rose, melissa).

Aromatic aldehydes are among the most powerful broad-spectrum anti-infectious and antibacterial compounds found in essential oils. They have moderately powerful antiviral, anti-fungal, and anti-parasitic functions, and moderately strong functions as immune system stimulants and general tonics. They are dermo-caustic and must be diluted appropriately.

Cinnamic aldehyde is an aromatic aldehyde with potent anti-microbial power. It is found in oils from Cinnamomum verum or zeylandicum (Ceylon cinnamon bark), Cinnamomum cassia (Chinese cinnamon bark), and Cinnamomum loureirii (Vietnamese cinnamon bark).

Other aromatic aldehydes are cuminal, found in Cuminum cyminum (cumin), and phellandral, found in Eucalyptus polybractea (blue mallee eucalyptus).

Ketones

Ketones are some of the most toxic of the compounds found in essential oils. However, some ketone-containing oils have excellent therapeutic value, although they are not generally considered strongly anti-microbial. Some oils containing ketones aid in wound healing and dissolving mucus, some are immune system stimulants, and some are anti-fungal. They can be used effectively in conjunction with stronger anti-microbial oils. Oils such as hyssop, eucalyptus and rosemary have moderate amounts of ketones; peppermint, spearmint, and rose geranium, which contain menthone, can be very beneficial when used properly.

Esters

Esters are not major anti-microbials, but they can be used in conjunction with stronger anti-microbial oils. Esters found in essential oils are normally very fragrant with a fruity aroma. Their therapeutic effects are balancing to the nervous system, calming, anti-inflammatory, and antispasmodic. An example of a well-known ester is linalyl acetate, which is found in lavender, clary sage, and petitgrain. Some esters also have anti-fungal and anti-microbial properties: geranium oil, which contains geranyl acetate, and helichrysum, which contains neryl acetate, possess anti-fungal properties; lemongrass oil, which contains geranyl acetate and linalyl acetate, has been found to be bactericidal against Helicobacter pylori (see below). These components are normally gentle in their actions and can be used with a wide safety margin.

Oxides

Oils containing oxides are generally camphoraceous in nature. As a group they are considered to have only mild anti-infectious effects, but they have excellent expectorant properties that can be used in conjunction with other oils. One of the most well-known of the non-toxic oxides is cineol (eucalyptol), which is found in eucalyptus and rosemary oils; these oils combine well with phenol-rich oils such as thyme and oregano for treatment of respiratory viral and bacterial infections.

In-vitro, In-vivo, and Clinical Testing

An extensive amount of documentation exists for in-vitro, in-vivo animal testing, and human clinical trials using essential oils. Below is a brief sample of some of these trials, to give a general overview of the range of possibilities that essential oils have for future clinical practice, including antibacterial, antiviral, and-fungal, and acaricidal.

Herpes Simplex

Essential oil of Melissa officinalis (lemon balm) was found to inhibit Herpes simplex virus type 2 (HSV-2), indicating that the oil contains an anti-HSV-2 substance.

(Antiviral activity of the volatile oils of Melissa officinalis L. against Herpes simplex virus type-2.; <u>Allahverdiyev A, Duran N, Ozguven M, Koltas S.</u>; Tropical Diseases Center, Faculty of Medicine, Cukurova University, Adana, Turkey.)

UTI

The antibacterial activity of essential oils extracted from Ocimum gratissimum (basil eugenol chemo-type), Cymbopogum citratus (lemon grass), and Salvia officinalis (sage) was assessed on bacterial strains derived from 100 urine samples. Salvia officinalis showed enhanced inhibitory activity, with 100 percent efficiency against Klebsiella and Enterobacter species, 96 percent against Escherichia coli, 83 percent against Proteus mirabilis, and 75 percent against Morganella morganii.

(Antibacterial activity of essential oils on microorganisms isolated from urinary tract infection; Rogério Santos Pereira; Tânia Cristina Sumita; Marcos Roberto Furlan; Antonio Olavo Cardoso Jorge; Mariko Ueno; Universidade de Taubaté. Taubaté, SP, Brasi)

Helicobacter pylori

Japanese researchers found that Cymbopogon citratus (lemongrass) and Lippia citriodora (lemon verbena) oils were bactericidal against Helicobacter pylori at 0.01 percent. In in-vivo studies, the density of H. pylori in the stomach of mice treated with lemongrass was significantly reduced compared with untreated mice. Resistance to lemongrass did not develop, whereas resistance to clarithromycin developed under the same conditions. The researchers concluded that the essential oils are bactericidal against H. pylori without the development of acquired resistance, and since resistance to antibiotics is emerging, that these essential oils may have potential as new and safe agents for inclusion in anti-H. pylori regimens.

(Antimicrobial activity of essential oils against Helicobacter pylori.; Ohno T, Kita M, Yamaoka Y, Imamura S, Yamamoto T, Mitsufuji S, Kodama T, Kashima K, Imanishi J.; Third Department of Internal Medicine, Kyoto Prefectural University of Medicine, Kyoto, 602-8566, Japan.)

Hepatitis

Fifty patients with chronic hepatitis C and ten with chronic hepatitis B were treated with essential oils such as ravensare, thyme, laurel, niaouli, and helichrysum, either in monotherapy or combined with standard allopathic drugs (interferon for hepatitis C). In patients with HCV treated with bitherapy and essential oils, tolerance and response to treatment was improved (80 percent good tolerance and 100 percent complete response especially for genotype 1). For patients with HCV treated with monotherapy (essential oils only), an improvement in hepatitis was noted in 64 percent of cases. For HBV, two cures were obtained with essential oils in monotherapy.

(The role of aromatherapy in the treatment of viral hepatitis; A.M. Giraud-Robert International Journal of Aromatherapy; Volume 15, Issue 4, 2005, Pages 183-192)

Oregano Oil Effective Again Shigella Dysentery

The results of this test showed that origanum volatile oil has obvious protective effect on mice infected with two strains of Shigella, and that it had germistatic and germicidal effects on dysentery bacteria. The researchers concluded that

Origanum volatile oil is an effective medicine against the infection of dysentery bacteria.

(Experimental study on the antibacterial effect of origanum volatile oil on dysentery bacilli in vivo and in vitro; Liao F, Huang Q, Yang Z, Xu H, Gao Q.; Department of Microbiology, Tongji Medical College, Huazhong University of Science and Technology, Wuhan 430030, China.)

Anti-Fungal (Tinea / Ringworm)

Japanese researchers conducing both in-vitro and in vivo experiments found that the essential oils of cinnamon bark, lemongrass, thyme, lavender, tea tree, and citronella oils (in increasing effectiveness) had potent anti-Trichophyton actions by vapor contact.

(In-vitro and in-vivo anti-Trichophyton activity of essential oils by vapour contact.; Inouye S, Uchida K, Yamaguchi H.; Teikyo University Institute of Medical Mycology, 359 Otsuka, Hachioji, Tokyo 192-03, Japan.)

Malodor of Tumor Necrosis

Oils of eucalyptus and tea tree have been found to be highly effective in removing the malodor of necrotic tumors in cancer patients, thereby improving the quality of life. Necrotic neoplastic ulcers are usually superinfected with anaerobic bacteria such as Bacteroides, Enterobacter, or Escherichia coli species. Additionally, these oils promote ulcer healing and re-epithelization. Adverse effects are uncommon and are usually limited to minor irritation at the time of application; the beneficial effects, however, have been quite pronounced.

(Antibacterial Essential Oils Reduce Tumor Smell and Inflammation in Cancer Patients; Journal of Clinical Oncology, Vol 23, No 7 (March 1), 2005: pp. 1588-a-1589)

Scabies

The acaricidal activity of Melaleuca alternifolia (tea tree) oil and some of its individual active components were tested on the itch mite Sarcoptes scabiei var hominis. A five per cent concentration of the oil was highly effective in reducing mite survival times, both in vitro and in vivo. The researchers suggest that because of increased resistance against anti-ectoparasitic compounds, tea tree oil has a potential role as a new topical acaricide, and confirm terpinen-4-ol as the primary active component.

(Acaricidal activity of Melaleuca alternifolia (tea tree) oil: in vitro sensitivity of sarcoptes scabiei var hominis to terpinen-4-ol.; <u>Walton SF, McKinnon M, Pizzutto S, Dougall A, Williams E, Currie BJ</u>.; Menzies School of Health Research, and Northern Territory Clinical School, Flinders University, Darwin, Australia.)

References

Determining the Antimicrobial Actions of Tea Tree Oil; Sean D. Cox, Cindy M. Mann, Julie L. Markham, John E. Gustafson, John R. Warmington and S. Grant Wyllie

Antiviral and Antimicrobial Properties of Essential Oils; Dominique Baudoux

<u>http://www.positivehealth.com/permit/Articles/Aromatherapy/baud55.htm</u>

http://www.ibms.org/index.cfm?method=science.general_science&subpage=-general_antimicrobial_effect_oils

Bioactivity of essential oils of selected temperate aromatic plants: antibacterial, antioxidant, antiinflammatory and other related pharmacological activities; Katya P Svoboda and Janice B Hampson; Plant Biology Department, SAC Auchincruive, Scotland, UK.

Terpenoids and Their Effects on Conifer Insects; Linda A. Mahaffey, Colorado State University; BI570 Spring 2004

Antimicrobial activity of the essential oil of Cestrum; Diurnum; Bhattacharjee I., Ghosh A. and Chandra G.; Mosquito Research Unit, Department of Zoology, The Burdwan University, India

Essential Oils Gain Credibility in the War on Pathogens; Marilyn Vail; <u>http://www.theida.com/pdf/MVailpaper.pdf</u>

Essential Oils - Nature's Powerful Anti-Viral Weapons; Melodie Kantner http://miqel.com/reading_library/archived_stories/essential-oil-infection-health.html

X

Helichrysum
Miracle Healing Oil

Introduction

Over the course of many years in clinical practice and involvement with the world of aromatherapy, I have seen and heard countless cases and testimonials of the healing benefits of essential oils. Of all the oils in the aromatic pharmacy and their multitude of therapeutic effects, I have come to appreciate Helichrysum italicum and its relatives as one of the most important and efficacious.

I had known for some time that this species was a valuable oil, but how important it was came into focus in a rather dramatic way last year at an aromatherapy training event. During the course of the program, which was attended by about two hundred fifty people, there were various testimonials about success stories with different oils and their preparations. When we came to helichrysum, however, the line to the microphone stretched across the room. The stories ranged from simple relief to dramatic cures, from home applications to post surgical hospital use, and in some cases to successes when allopathic treatments and drugs had failed. It was for this reason that my respect for this unusual oil increased, and I now rank it as one of the most important oils for both home and clinical use.

Etymology

There are two explanations of the origin of the word helichrysum: one is that the name is derived from the Greek word helisso, meaning "to turn around," and the second is that it is derived from the Greek Helios, the personification of the sun; both concur that chrysos refers to its golden color.

Botany

Members of the Asteraceae family, there are over 600 species of Helichrysum occurring worldwide; a number of these are rare and endangered. Helichrysum italicum, the most important essential oil producing species, grows in the Mediterranean region. It is a drought tolerant evergreen shrub found in dry, sandy and stony areas, which flowers from May to August. There are a number of subspecies of H. italicum, including ssp. italicum, ssp. microphyllum, and ssp. serotinum.

Helichrysum italicum Essential Oil

Numerous references can be found to traditional uses of roots, leaves and flowers of different helichrysum species around the world for a wide range of applications. The therapeutic actions of many of these, especially those that utilize the flowers, are probably based on the essential oil constituents. For the purpose of this article, we will focus specifically on the essential oil of H. italicum.

The essential oil of H. italicum is most concentrated in the flowering tops during the months of June and July, when they give off a delectable herbaceous honey-sweet aroma; Napoleon famously remarked that he could smell the island of Corsica before sighting it, so rich was the fragrance of the landscape.

Helichrysum italicum is one of the more expensive oils on the market, especially the true Corsican variety. A number of factors contribute to this, including crop failures in recent years and a low yield of approximately .1% oil from biomass, meaning that one ton of flowers yields about one kilo of essential oil. The oil is typically steam distilled from the flowers.

Chemistry

The bright yellow flower heads contain principally essential oils, flavonoids (helichrysin A and B) and tannins.

The essential oils of different helichrysum species vary widely in constituents; the oils of H. italicum vary depending on the origin, frequency of harvesting and soil chemistry. In general the H. italicum oils are composed primarily of monoterpenes such as pinene, camphene, myrcene, and limonene, and monoterpene-derived alcohols such as linalool, teripinene-4-ol, nerol, and geraniol. Nerol and its ester neryl acetate are also primary compounds that are attributed to the healing powers of the oil. A number of sesquiterpenes are also present, such as selinene and curcumene, as well as a number of diketones.

I have had five species of helichrysum essential oils tested using gas chromatography, to distinguish the differences in their compounds. The following is a short summation of the most prevalent compounds and a short review of their therapeutic significance.

Helichrysum italicum, Croatia
α-PINENE: 23.47%

LIMONENE: 4.23%
1,8-CINEOLE: 2.63%
ITALICENE: 3.07%
β-CARYOPHYLLENE: 6.12%
γ-CURCUMENE: 8.26%
NERYL ACETATE: 12.09%
β-SELINENE: 2.81%
α-SELINENE: 2.52%
α-CURCUMENE: 2.92%
GERANIOL: 2.29%
ITALIDIONE I: 2,96%
ITALIDIONE II: .79%
ITALIDIONE III: .91%

One of the key ingredients that determines the quality of H. italicum oil is neryl acetate. The percentage ranges from less than seven percent to over forty, with the Corsican strains having a uniquely high level because of climate and soil condition. While not an expert in the subject, I would surmise that this sample from Croatia could be considered a mid-grade oil from the standpoint of this particular compound, as well as having somewhat low levels of italidione, which gives the oil its typical fragrance; it appears to have relatively normal levels of the sesquiterpenes caryophyllene and curcumene.

Helichrysum gymnocephalum, South Africa
α-PINENE: 4.17%
β-PINENE: 3.27%
1,8-CINEOLE: 70.08%
p-CYMENE: 4.04%
TERPINENE-4-OL: 2.84%

Helichrysum bractiferum, South Africa
α-PINENE: 4.93%
β-PINENE: 12.40%
LIMONENE: 3.05%
1,8-CINEOLE: 27.38%
β-CARYOPHYLLENE: 9.44%
α-HUMULENE: 10.75%

Helichrysum odoritisimum, South Africa
α-PINENE: 28.24%
1,8-CINEOLE: 28.24%
β-CARYOPHYLLENE: 8.51%
δ-CADINENE: 3.91%
γ-CADINENE: 3.36%

Helichrysum splendidum, South Africa
α-PINENE: 2.36%
β-PINENE: 8.33%
1,8-CINEOLE: 14.60%
β-BOURBONENE: 2.89%
GERMACRENE D: 7.71%
α-MUUROLENE: 2.30%
BICYCLOGERMACRENE: 2.80%
δ-CADINENE: 13.53%
γ-CADINENE: 4.02%

With varying levels of 1,8 cineole (eucalyptol), and pinenes as primary compounds, these species from South Africa could be considered similar to eucalyptus or conifer oils with respiratory decongestant, expectorant and mucus membrane antimicrobial effects; traditional uses of the leaves and flowers of different species include chest complaints, coughs, colds, and fevers.

Therapeutic Applications

Injuries

One of helichrysum's most valuable and consistently cited benefits is for treatment of bruising and swelling from soft tissue injuries. Its anti-coagulant and blood-vitalizing powers minimize tissue reactions to contusions such as constriction of blood flow and subsequent damage to cells. The oil has pronounced anti-spasmotic and anti-inflammatory effects, which in turn produce pain-relieving analgesic benefits. In this sense the oil could be compared to arnica, although I would personally rate helichrysum as more effective. It can be applied undiluted and frequently without concern of dermotoxicity, or combined with arnica-infused oil.

Scar Tissue

Helichrysum rates among the best essential oils for resolving scar tissue, both new and old. I have found this effect to be accentuated when it is combined with frankincense oil. Both oils are sometimes referred to as cictarizants, meaning they assist wound healing by forming scar tissue; helichrysum has been found effective in clinical trials for closing open wounds and promoting rapid tissue healing. In this case, however, these two oils could be termed the opposite in the sense that once the scar tissue is formed they help break it down and restore normal healthy skin. The mechanisms for this in the case of helichrysum appear to be the oil's ability to increase cutaneous microcirculation, a high level of antioxidant activity, its support of increased collagen production, and enhancement of vascular endothelial growth factor (VEGF); the latter is a signal protein produced by cells that stimulates vasculogenesis and angiogenesis that is part of the system which restores oxygen supply to tissues when blood circulation is inadequate.

Cosmetic

Among the essential oils, helichrysum is unparalleled in its anti-inflammatory, cell regenerating and tissue healing properties, which can be explained by the same physiological activities that heal scars. As an anti-oxidant with collagen-increasing virtues it is renowned for restoring aging and wrinkled skin. It has purifying, cleansing, and antiseptic functions on the skin, and is attributed with hydrating and rejuvenating powers for cells of the stratum corneum. A vital component of cosmetic skin care formulations, regular use reduces broken capillaries, stretch marks, and age spots. Other skin conditions including burns, acne, allergies, dermatitis, eczema, inflammation, and warts may be improved by application of this oil.

Anti-inflammatory

Along with its ability to reduce pain and speed healing of injuries, helichrysum has significant anti-inflammatory powers. It is specifically useful for direct and undiluted application to arthritic joints.

Respiratory

The oil of H. italicum can be inhaled directly from the palms, with steam, or used in a diffuser for its antimicrobial benefits in the respiratory system. It is mucolytic and expectorant and decongestant. These effects could be attributed primarily to the presence of monoterpenes such as pinene.

Neurological

Aromatherapists consider helichrysum to have a tonifying effect on the nervous system when used in diffusers or direct palm inhalation, with stress-reducing and mood-uplifting effects.

Other anecdotal stories are told of cases of tinnitus that have improved from the use of helichrysum oil on a cotton ball placed in the ear. I have personally seen a handful of such cases and can confirm this effect, which I would attribute to the oil's anti-inflammatory, microcirculation-enhancing, decongesting and antimicrobial powers at work on underlying associated causes.

I have also heard rumors that the oil has a stimulating effect on hair growth, which could be attributed to its powers to increase cutaneous circulation and thereby increase nourish, rejuvenate and detoxify hair follicles.

Helichrysum Oil Recipes:

Scar blend: 12 drops Helichrysum italicum, 6 drops carrot seed oil, 6 drops Rosemary verbenone in 15 ml rosehip seed and tamanu oil

Inflammation blend: 8 drops Helichrysum italicum, 8 drops German chamomile oil, neat or diluted in calendula-infused olive oil.

A Sampling of Research Studies on Helichrysum italicum

Anti-inflammatory and antioxidant properties of Helichrysum italicum
The anti-inflammatory and antioxidant activities of the aerial part of Helichrysum italicum extracts have been established in various in-vivo and in-vitro experimental models. We conclude that the anti-inflammatory activity of Helichrysum italicum can be explained by multiple effects, including inflammatory enzyme inhibition, free-radical scavenging activity and corticoid-like effects. (J Pharm Pharmacol. 2002 Mar;54(3):365-71.)

Assessment of the anti-inflammatory activity and free radical scavenger activity of tiliroside.
Three flavonoids, gnaphaliin, pinocembrin and tiliroside, isolated from Helichrysum italicum, were studied in vitro for their antioxidant and/or scavenger properties and in vivo in different models of inflammation. However, only tiliroside significantly reduced the oedema and leukocyte infiltration. As in the case of other flavonoids, the anti-inflammatory activity of tiliroside could be based on its antioxidant properties, although other mechanisms are probably involved. (Eur J Pharmacol. 2003 Feb 7;461(1):53-61.)

Helichrysum italicum extract interferes with the production of enterotoxins by Staphylococcus aureus.
CONCLUSIONS: H. italicum interferes with growth and production of enterotoxins by Staph. aureus. SIGNIFICANCE AND IMPACT OF THE STUDY: There is considerable interest in the use of natural compounds as alternative methods to control undesirable pathogenic micro-organisms.
(Lett Appl Microbiol. 2002;35(3):181-4.)

Effects of Helichrysum italicum extract on growth and enzymatic activity of Staphylococcus aureus.
H. italicum extract had an inhibitory effect on S. aureus strains reducing both their growth and some of the enzymes such as coagulase, DNAse, thermonuclease and lipase. Helichrysum italicum extract could be a novel antimicrobial agent, less toxic to human skin and tissues, worthy of further studies.
(Int J Antimicrob Agents. 2001 Jun;17(6):517-20.)

Arzanol, a prenylated heterodimeric phloroglucinyl pyrone, inhibits eicosanoid biosynthesis and exhibits anti-inflammatory efficacy in vivo.
Based on its capacity to inhibit in vitro HIV-1 replication in T cells and the release of pro-inflammatory cytokines in monocytes, the prenylated heterodimeric phloroglucinyl α-pyrone arzanol was identified as the major anti-inflammatory and anti-viral constituent from Helichrysum italicum. Taken together, our data show that arzanol potently inhibits the biosynthesis of pro-inflammatory lipid mediators like PGE(2)in vitro and in vivo, providing a mechanistic rationale for the anti-inflammatory activity of H. italicum, and a rationale for further pre-clinical evaluation of this novel anti-inflammatory lead.
(Biochem Pharmacol. 2011 Jan 15;81(2):259-68. Epub 2010 Oct 8.)

Arzanol, an anti-inflammatory and anti-HIV-1 phloroglucinol alpha-Pyrone from Helichrysum italicum ssp. microphyllum.
Arzanol inhibited HIV-1 replication in T cells and the release of pro-inflammatory cytokines in LPS-stimulated primary monocytes, qualifying as a novel plant-derived anti-inflammatory and antiviral chemotype worth further investigation.
(J Nat Prod. 2007 Apr;70(4):608-12. Epub 2007 Feb 22.)

Protective role of arzanol against lipid peroxidation in biological systems.
The results of the work qualify arzanol as a potent natural antioxidant with a protective effect against lipid oxidation in biological systems.
(Chem Phys Lipids. 2011 Jan;164(1):24-32. Epub 2010 Oct 7.)

Evaluation of antiherpesvirus-1 and genotoxic activities of Helichrysum italicum extract.
The antiherpes virus-1 and genotoxic activities of diethyl ether extract from flowering tops of Helichrysum italicum (Compositae) were investigated. The extract showed significant antiviral activity at concentrations ranging from 400 to 100 microg/ml. This activity was not due to cytotoxic effect of the extract since Vero cells exhibited altered morphology or growth characteristics indicative of cytotoxic effects at higher concentration (800 microg/ml). Moreover H. italicum extract showed no DNA-damaging activity at concentrations up to 2000 microg/disk.
(New Microbiol. 2003 Jan;26(1):125-8.)

Chemical composition, plant genetic differences, and antifungal activity of the essential oil of Helichrysum italicum G. Don ssp. microphyllum (Willd) Nym.
The chemical composition of the essential oil of the Sardinian dwarf curry plant [Helichrysum italicum G. Don ssp. microphyllum (Willd) Nym] was studied. Genetic analysis suggested the presence of two chemotypes; morphological and chemical differences confirmed the presence of two chemotypes (A and B). The maximum yields were 0.18 and 0.04% (v/w) for flowering tops and stems, respectively. The concentrations of nerol and its esters (acetate and propionate), limonene, and linalool reach their highest values during the flowering stage both in flowers and in stems. Besides the essential oil, type B showed an interesting antifungal activity.
J Agric Food Chem. 2003 Feb 12;51(4):1030-4.

Chemical and biological studies on two Helichrysum species of Greek origin.
The chemical composition of the essential oils obtained from the aerial parts of Helichrysum amorginum and H.italicum were analysed with GC and GC/MS. From the twenty-five identified constituents representing the 89.98% and 82.06% of the two oils respectively, geraniol, geranyl acetate, neryl acetate, and nerolidol were the major components. Furthermore, it was found that the oils exhibited definite antibacterial activity against the six tested Gram (+/-) bacteria.
Planta Med. 1996 Aug;62(4):377-9.

XI

Roses

A Short Timeline of Roses

Thirty-five million years ago: Fossil records indicate the first appearance of roses.
3000 BCE: The first cultivation of roses. Ancient China and Persia are historically believed to be the regions where roses were first cultivated.

1000 BCE: The earliest known written reference to roses growing in a garden is a Sumerian record found at the Mesopotamian city of Ur, in what is now Iraq.

69-30 BCE: Cleopatra carpets the floor of her palace with rose petals.

Roman Empire: Roses are cultivated extensively throughout the Middle East. Roman nobility establish large public rose gardens in the south of Rome.

AD 170: From the tomb of Hawara on Crete comes a wreath that is the oldest preserved rose species.

10th – 17th Centuries: The rose industry is developed and dominated by Persia. In this period Baghdad is famous for its rose gardens.

12th and 13th century: European Crusaders bring back specimens of either Rosa damascena or Rosa gallica from their travels to the Middle East. Roses become highly valued in monasteries of Old Europe. One of the oldest garden roses, Rosa gallica officinalis, the "Apothecary rose," is considered capable of curing a multitude of illnesses.

1455–1489: War of the Roses. The rose is used as a symbol for the factions fighting to control England: the red rose of Lancaster and the white rose of York.

15th -16th century: Turkish merchants import Rosa damascena for cultivation throughout the Balkan countries, establishing the "Valley of Roses" in Bulgaria in the region of Kazanlik, meaning "the place of stills."

1597: Fourteen varieties of roses are officially recognized in Europe.

1629: Twenty-four varieties are recognized.

1800: The first red rose arrives in Europe from China. Previously, all European roses such as Rosa damascena were pink or white.

Mid - late 18th century: Introduction of cultivated roses into Europe from China; by the end of that century there are over 1,000 varieties. Most modern roses can be traced back to this ancestry.

19th century: Centered in the "Valley of Roses," the Bulgarian rose oil industry reigns as a near-monopoly of the world market.

1867: The modern era of rose hybrids begins with the development of the first hybrid tea rose.

1900: Rose breeders create yellow and orange roses after the discovery of a wild mutant yellow flower.

1960's: Discovery and analysis of trace constituents of rose oil responsible for its fragrance. The rose ketones beta-Damascenone and beta-Damascone become two of the most important chemicals in the fragrance and flavoring industries.

Present: There are over 30,000 varieties of roses.

The Cultivation, Harvesting and Distillation of Roses

Roses belong to the Rosaceae family, which contains three to four thousand species in about one hundred twenty genera. This botanic family includes apples, pears, strawberries and raspberries. Roses have the most complicated family tree of any known flower species.

Of the thousands of varieties of roses, only a few give the fragrance sought by perfumeries. The pink-red Rosa damascena forma triginipetala (Damask rose) is the primary species grown in Bulgaria's Valley of Roses. The white Rosa damascena var. alba is a hardier species that is sometimes planted around the Damask roses. The Damask rose is the most important, as it yields a higher quantity of oil which is considered to be a superior quality. Rosa centifolia and Rosa bourbonica are cultivated and distilled in India.

Most rose cultivation for distillation purposes is done on small family-owned farms, and is typically part of a diverse intercropping with other crops. This is true in all major rose growing regions including Bulgaria, Turkey, Morocco, and India. For example, the rose farm and distillery I visited in Rajasthan grows roses intercropped with vegetables for the local market and various medicinal and fruit trees such as amla (Emblica officinalis) and varieties of mangoes. Because vast quantities of roses are required to produce small amounts of oil, distilleries are cooperatively operated.

In the Valley of Roses, the harvest season begins with the opening of the flowers around the second week of May, and usually lasts three to four weeks. Hot dry weather reduces the yield and length of the season, while cooler moister weather increases them.

The oil content of the flowers is highest around two in the morning. Harvesting begins before sunrise and typically ends in the middle morning. The harvesting should be done while the dew is still on the petals, as there is a considerable loss of volatile oil content in the flowers due to evaporation by the suns rays.

Bags of roses are transported to the nearest still as quickly as possible, as the flowers begin to deteriorate immediately.

Rose *otto* is the essential oil extracted from Rosa damascena. The term otto is thought to be a derivative of the word *attar*, which specifically refers to the Indian method of distilling botanical fragrances into a base of sandalwood oil.

Distillation of rose otto proceeds in two stages. The first distillation produces the first hydrosol and a layer of thick brown oil, which is extremely concentrated and valuable. After separating the oil the hydrosol is then redistilled to extract the remaining oil within it, producing a second hydrosol and oil. The two oils are then blended to produce rose otto, while the hydrosol is sold as rose water.

The fresh rose otto must be aged to bring out its best aroma; this can take up to a year. The fragrance will continue to improve if stored properly.

1,000 kilos of flowers (one metric ton) consists of approximately 400,000 individual flowers. It takes around 3,500 kilos of flowers to produce one kilo of oil. Hence it takes 1,400,000 handpicked blossoms to produce thirty-five ounces of oil. It takes 40,000 blossoms to make one ounce of oil, and sixty-seven blossoms to make one drop of oil.

A well managed rose garden produces from 1,250-1,650 kilos of flowers per acre. Thus, it requires two to three acres of land to produce one kilo of oil. However, the yield of oil depends on the climate, time of the harvest, condition of the flowers and the method of distillation.

Therapeutic Uses of Roses and Rose Oil

Roses and rose oil have a vast number of therapeutic applications and more are emerging through ongoing research. Besides its role as a major ingredient of perfumery, rose oil has a history of medicinal use dating back at least five thousand years, yet some of its most important constituents have only been discovered recently.

It has been known for over a hundred years that the main constituent of rose oil's over two hundred seventy five compounds is citronellol. In the 1960's and 70's researchers began reporting the trace constituents of rose oil, with beta-Damascenone being the most important.

Although Damascenone constitutes only a minor percentage of rose oil, it contributes the maximum percentage of fragrance. Citronellol, although it can be found in concentrations as high as thirty-eight percent of the oil, has only four percent of relative odor units, or fragrance presence in the oil. On the other hand, Damascenone has over seventy percent of the perceivable odor units of the oil, with only .1 percent concentration in the oil. (An "odor unit" value is determined by dividing the concentration of a component [in ppb] by the component's detection threshold level [in ppb].)

Beta-Damascenone and another rose ketone, beta-Damascone, are two of the most important chemicals in the fragrance and flavoring industries. Citronellol and Damascenone are responsible for many of the rose oil's therapeutic properties.

In Ayurvedic terms roses and rose oil are considered *sattvic*, meaning that they have a compassionate quality that harms no one; *tridoshic*, meaning that they benefit all body types; *pitta pacifying*, meaning that they have cooling and anti-inflammatory properties; *ojas building*, meaning that they rejuvenate immunity by building nutritional essence; and supportive to *shukra*, meaning that they increase semen and reproductive fluids.

Ayurvedic medicine uses rose oil both topically and orally for treating a variety of inflammatory conditions, either as a single remedy or prepared with other herbs or minerals. An infusion of petals is a mild remedy for pitta symptoms such as headaches, throat inflammation and hangovers. Pearl *pisti* is a cooling anti-inflammatory compound prepared by triturating rose oil with pearl powder and then exposing the mixture to the rays of the full moon.

Rosewater can be used safely for inflammation and infections of the eyes such as conjunctivitis, and as a douche for vaginal infections and inflammation. It is helpful as a mouthwash for gingivitis, and safe for children while teething. Rose honey has also been used traditionally for reducing inflammatory conditions.

The anti-inflammatory effects of rose are possibly due to beta-Damascenone's anti-spasmotic effects on vascular tissue, which has been found to have potency in the same range as papaverine. (1)

Rose oil has been found to be a potent inhibitor of Helicobacter pylori, and is thought to exert a sanitizing effect in the gut. Its antibiotic effect extends to plants as well and is a potential agent for controlling infections in commercial crops such as tomatoes. (2) Aromatherapy writers advise applying rose oil undiluted on shingles for its antiviral properties.

Aromatherapy writers have stated that rose oil has a pronounced effect on the circulatory system, that it promotes circulation, cleanses the blood, relieves heart congestion, and tones the capillaries. One study validating this claim found that a capsule containing sixty-eight milligrams of Bulgarian rose oil, 30,000 IU vitamin A and 250 milligrams sunflower seed oil administered twice daily before meals for one hundred ten days had a marked hypolipidemic effect and reduced arterial hypertension. The remedy was tolerated well, with no side effects or contraindications for its use. (3)

Roses and rose oil have a long history of symbolic association with love, devotion, passion and spirituality, a paradox expressed by its sensual flower protected by thorns. Sacred scents such as rose that are evocative of spiritual and erotic moods have always been used for their uplifting effects on the heart and emotions. Rose oil in particular has a long history of use as a gentle but potent antidepressant. It seems particularly beneficial for sensitive people who are emotionally overwhelmed, and for those suffering grief and sadness. It reduces anxiety and melancholy. Being the queen of flowers, as well as an extremely precious oil, it supports higher self esteem.

Rose oil is used in Ayurveda as a rejuvenating aphrodisiac. Rose attar, which is prepared by distilling rose petals into a base of sandalwood oil, is considered a specific remedy for depletion of semen that works by relaxing the adrenals and sympathetic nervous system; it is used in massage for this purpose.

Rose oil has traditionally been viewed as having anti-stress properties with calmative, relaxant and mood-enhancing effects. It is used as a mild sedative that is soothing to the nervous system, and considered valuable for conditions of nervous stress that affect the circulatory and digestive. Rose oil inhalation produced an anxiolytic-like effect similar to diazepam in adult male rats. (4) The pharmacologically active constituents that produced rose oil's anti-anxiety-like effect have been determined to be 2-phenethyl alcohol and citronellol. (5) Inhalation of rose oil decreases sympathetic activity and adrenaline concentrations in normal adult subjects. (6)

Roses have numerous beneficial effects in the digestive system, and offer many nutritional benefits as well. The petals are mildly laxative, and used in syrups for constipation. The fruits of many species are rich in vitamins and minerals, especially vitamins A, C and E, flavonoids and other bioactive compounds. Rose oil has high concentrations of the essential lipid linoleic acid, which has been found to have anti-tumor effects.

Gulkand, rose petal jam, is an exquisite Ayurvedic nutritive tonic made from fresh rose petals, sugar cane juice and rejuvenating herbs. It is used as a cooling tonic that treats malnutrition, liver weakness, anemia, chronic fatigue, biliousness and acidity, and a wide variety of other deficiency conditions. It can be used by all constitutional types, and is especially good for vata and pitta.

Rose oil is one of the least toxic of the essential oils, which makes it ideal for massage and skin care; it is safely used in dilution for baby oil. Rose oil is a valuable ingredient of cosmetics. It has a healing influence for every skin type, especially infected, inflamed, dry, and sensitive skin (pitta and vata). Rosewater is an excellent for the same types of skin problems. Rosehip seed oil, extracted from the seeds of Rosa mosqueta, is one of the best anti-inflammatory emollient oils for dry and inflamed conditions of the skin such as eczema.

References

(1) (Antispasmodic activity of beta-damascenone and E-phytol isolated from Ipomoea pes-caprae. Pongprayoon U, Baeckstrom P, Jacobsson U, Lindstrom M, Bohlin L. Department of Pharmacognosy, Uppsala University, Sweden.)

(2) (Antibacterial activity of Rosa damascena essential oil. Basim E, Basim H. University of Suleyman Demirel, Faculty of Agriculture, Department of Plant Protection, Isparta, Turkey.)

(3) (Girosital. Clinical trial in primary hyperlipoproteinaemia.

Kirov M, Koev P, Popiliev I, Apostolov I, Marinova V Medico Biologic Information)

(4) (Anxiolytic-like effects of rose oil inhalation on the elevated plus-maze test in rats. de Almeida RN, Motta SC, de Brito Faturi C, Catallani B, Leite JR. Department of Physiology and Pathology/LTF, Universidade Federal da Paraiba-Caixa, P.O. Box 5009, PB 58051-970, Joao Pessoa, Brazil)

(5) (Anticonflict effects of rose oil and identification of its active constituents. Umezu T, Ito H, Nagano K, Yamakoshi M, Oouchi H, Sakaniwa M, Morita M. Endocrine Disruptors and Dioxin Project Group, Japan)

(6) (Effects of fragrance inhalation on sympathetic activity in normal adults. Haze S, Sakai K, Gozu Y. Product Development Center, Shiseido Co., Ltd., Hayabuchi, Yokohama, Japan)

XII

Frankincense and Myrrh
The Botany, Culture, and Therapeutic Uses of the World's Two Most Important Resins

Introduction

Frankincense and myrrh are without a doubt the world's two most important resins. Although other resins, such as pine, copal, styrax, and dragon blood have played important roles in ethnobotanical medicine, none have been as widely distributed and universally utilized, as economically important, or so highly regarded. This paper presents an overview of these valuable trees and the history, culture, and some of the medical uses of their resins.

Ancient Frankincense and Myrrh Trade

The earliest history of frankincense and myrrh trade is shrouded in myth. The gum-bearing trees were said to be guarded by fierce red snakes which leaped into the air to inflict fatal bites on any intruder. The trees were be- lieved to grow in forbidding mountain areas surrounded by swirling mists that caused deadly diseases and fatal epidemics. Frankincense and myrrh brought from such inhospitable terrain was considered to be sacred to the gods, and reserved for divine worship.

The frankincense and myrrh market of the Old World was highly lucrative for almost 1,500 years. The source was based in a small geographic area, the demand far exceeded the trees' ability to produce, and there were great difficulties in delivering the materials over vast distances. As a result, the flow of these resins as commodi- ties made the Arabs who dealt in them among the wealthiest on earth at the time.

The trading of frankincense and myrrh expanded greatly around the 11th century BCE, with the establishing of improved land routes and domestication of the camel. From the harvesting centers in northeastern Africa and the Arabian Peninsula, the resin was transported to Egypt, and then by sea to India and other destinations. The life of the Arabian frankincense and myrrh merchant was one of camel caravans crossing barren sands, navigating by stars, and following a route between secret water cisterns hidden from roaming thieves. Many cities, such as the rock-carved canyon city of Petra, prospered and reached high levels of sophisticated civilization because of the wealth brought by these resins. By 1000 BCE, myrrh and frankincense were widely distributed throughout the Old World. Babylon, Assyria, Egypt, Persia, Rome, Greece, and China all imported these resins, to be used as temple incenses and as important medicines. Frankincense and myrrh were prized possessions in the ancient world, rivaling the value of many precious gems and metals.

The height of the frankincense trade occurred during the second century CE when some three thousand tons were shipped each year from south Arabia to Greece, Rome and the Mediterranean region. After the 3rd century CE the trade went into its decline, although demand still supported Arabia for another three hundred years. Even into the Middle Ages frankincense was an Arabian trading commodity.

Economic and Ecological Value

Frankincense and myrrh trees are crucial for preservation of fragile desert ecologies, and are a source of sustainable livelihood for local societies, especially those maintaining nomadic and semi-nomadic lifestyles. Many of the ecological, economic, and spiritual traditions surrounding these trees are in danger of being lost. Large areas of their native habitat have been cleared for cultivation, firewood, building materials, and animal fodder. Without the trees, wind and rain erode the underlying soil, producing infertile sub-desert conditions and forcing people to migrate to cities. However, if protected, these trees could provide valuable crops of oils, gums and resins, as well as preserve traditional agrarian lifestyles.

The early frankincense trade was of great economic significance to those who lived in the areas where the trees grew, to those who managed the trade in the various market outlets, and to those who controlled the overland trade routes. For the semi-nomadic people living off the land, harvesting of frankincense has historically proven to be a viable livelihood. The harvesting of the resins is a sustainable practice, whereas the current harvesting of the wood is not.

In Somalia, which is one of the poorest and least-developed countries in the world, trials to plant new stands of frankincense are currently underway. Current interest in frankincense essential oil in the West has helped develop a small but strong market for Somali frankincense. While destruction threatens some species of Boswellia in some regions, in others there is an abundance that is not being utilized. Ethiopia and Sudan are the biggest exporters of Boswellia papyrifera, with abundant supplies of this type of resin offering good potential for economic development in these countries.

Frankincense

Origin of the Name

The Arabs called the milky sap of the frankincense tree al lubán, from the word for milk. The same word gave rise to the name of Lebanon, whose mountains were always capped by milky snow. Al lubán became anglicized to olibanum, which is another name for frankincense. The word frankincense means the true, or frank, incense.

Origin and Habitat

Frankincense trees are found in Oman, Somalia, Ethiopia, Yemen, the southern Arabian Peninsula, and India. The desert of the Dhofar region in southern Oman is the source of Boswellia sacra, "sacred frankincense." The Boswellia serrata, Indian frankincense, is widely distributed and abundant in the dry, hilly parts of India. The trees on the Somali coast grow out of polished marble rocks without soil; the purer the marble the stronger the tree. The Boswellia papyrifera grows primarily in Ethiopia and Sudan.

Botany and Morphology of Frankincense

Frankincense is the hardened oleo gum resin exudate (a mixture of volatile oil, gum, and resin) from different species of Boswellia. It is a translucent, brittle, whitish-yellow substance, in roundish, club-shaped, pear-shaped, or irregular tears, and usually covered by a whitish substance produced by the pieces rubbing against each other. The purer varieties are almost colorless, whitish, or with a greenish tinge, and easily flammable. It has a sub-acrid, terebinthinate, bitter, and aromatic taste. It melts with difficulty, becomes soft and adhesive by chewing, and forms an incomplete white emulsion when rubbed up with water.

When burned, frankincense produces a brilliant flame and diffuses an agreeable aroma. This aroma is described as fresh, balsamic, dry, resinous, slightly green, with a fruit topnote and a diffusive note of unripe apple peel. This fragrance is due predominantly to mixtures of complex mono- and sesquiterpenes.

There are approximately twenty-five species in the genus. The major species are Boswellia sacra (synonymous with Boswellia carteri), Boswellia papyrifera, Boswellia serrata (Indian frankincense), Boswellia thurifera, Boswellia neglecta, and Boswellia frereana.

There is much confusion surrounding the proper identification of the various types of frankincense found in the market. Contributing to this confusion are differences in species, varieties of individual species, effects of microclimates on the trees, variations in quality of harvested resin, and time of harvesting. To those who gather the resin in the wild, these differences are not economically important enough to differentiate between species. Wild-harvested frankincense therefore has unique individual characteristics.

In the Dhofar region the trees tend to be short and squat, reaching a height of five meters, with papery peeling bark which varies from white to reddish in color. Multiple trunks often rise out of a cushion or disk-like base which helps stabilize the tree on the boulders and steep embankments where they grow. Alternate, pinnately compound leaves cluster at the end of branches. Small white to pale pink flowers appear on the tree from September to November and are followed by small capsule, obovoid type fruits. All parts of the tree from the flowers, fruit, bark, and wood, are charged with the resinous perfume.

The Indian Frankincense (Boswellia Serrata) is a large, tall, deciduous tree having a straight, buttressed trunk with a clear bole and widespread branches. The trunk and branch bark are gray in color and have hard, sharp, and conical spines.

Frankincense trees can live for at least a hundred years. Their flowers are popular with bees.

Harvesting

In Oman, frankincense is gathered by Bedouins; trees are owned by the families living in a particular area where they grow. The guardianship of the trees is passed on from generation to generation, and there are ancient rituals surrounding the harvesting of the resin. On the southern Arabian coast, the trees are tapped yearly by visiting parties of Somalis, who pay the Arabs for the privilege of collecting frankincense.

Frankincense from Oman is harvested during the spring and fall, with that produced from the fall harvest considered the best. In India, the collecting of Boswellia serrata resin, or Salai-guggul, is carried out towards the end of October.

The general process of harvesting frankincense is similar in the various regions. The trees are scored at various places along the main trunk and branches with a sharp metal blade, or by scraping away a portion of the bark. The wounds in the bark produce milky white resin, which hardens as it dries on the tree. Healthy and mature trees are selected for tapping, and proper tapping does not injure the tree. The oleo gum resin secreted from the cortex is fragrant, transparent, and golden yellow and solidifies into brownish-yellow tears or drops. In India, the oleo gum resin is scraped and collected in a circular tray placed around the trunk. In Oman, once the season's collection is completed, the raw frankincense is stored in dry caves to cure before being sold.

In general, there are four grades of frankincense tears. The first is the "superfine," which is translucent, very light yellow and free from impurities. The second is "first quality," which is brownish yellow and less translucent, but free from impurities and bark. The third is "second quality," which is brownish, semi translucent, and containing some impurities. The lowest grade is "third quality," which is dark brown, opaque, and with impurities. In India, the highest grade is what is collected first, while in Oman the later collections are considered superior.

When the oleo gum resin is collected exclusively for essential oil production the fresh semi-solid material is used. It is not allowed to dry, because drying would cause many trace components to be lost.

Essential Oil

The essential oil of frankincense contains more than two hundred molecular compounds, which give the essence a very complex bouquet and range of therapeutic applications. Even within a particular species of tree there can be considerable difference in the proportion of these components depending on the microclimate and soil where the trees grow, the season at which the resin is harvested, and a number of other variables. The oil is also influenced by age and storage. Frankincense oils are therefore diverse from an olfactory and therapeutic standpoint.

Traditional Uses of Resin

Large amounts of frankincense tears are consumed in the local harvesting areas. The fresh gum is chewed for strengthening the teeth and gums, to stimulate digestion, to expel congested phlegm, and to combat halitosis. Small pieces of gum are inserted into painful teeth and to combat dental caries. The resin is boiled in milk until a thick paste is formed, which is then applied as a poultice to inflamed swellings such as mastitis, and taken internally for bronchial conditions. It is infused in wine for respiratory conditions, and in Saudi Arabia the gum is added to coffee.

In the Dhofar region, women smooth the soft gum over their hair to keep it in place and give it a shiny appearance. Cones of the resin are burned as candles outdoors at night to keep away wild animals and evil spirits. The ancient Egyptians used frankincense and myrrh for embalming, as resins are bacteriostatic and do not decay. Frankincense is used in Arab homes to perfume clothes and purify the atmosphere. It is used in traditional festivities such as weddings and religious celebrations. Visitors are often offered bowls of burning frankincense; men use it to fumigate their beards, while women perfume their head shawls. Students facing exams place two or three of the highest quality tears in water with a piece of iron overnight and drink the resulting liquid first thing in the morning; this has been found to improve their memory and consequent chances of success.

Therapeutic Properties

The oleo gum resins produced by trees such as frankincense, myrrh, pine, spruce, fir, and others are a major part of the trees' immune system. Tree sap has antibiotic and antifungal properties that protect the tree from infections, wound-healing properties for closing and regenerating the bark, and pheromone-like signaling mechanisms for repelling insect attackers and attracting the attacker's natural predators. When humans use oleo gum resins or essential oils derived from trees, we are utilizing the molecular components of the trees' immune system to boost our own. The general functions of frankincense resin and essential oil can therefore be described as immune-enhancing; antibiotic, antifungal, antiviral, and antiseptic; and wound-healing, with pronounced anti-inflammatory properties. Below is a brief list of the most important therapeutic applications of frankincense, which is by no means complete; the uses of frankincense are so numerous that it can accurately be described as a panacea, used for everything from colds to cancers. Since the resin is widely used for chewing, it can be assumed that it is not toxic to humans; however, use of the essential oil must be guided by appropriate precautions.

Skin

Frankincense has cytophylactic properties, meaning that it encourages healthy growth and regeneration of skin cells. Because it has rejuvenating and wound-healing effects on the skin, it is useful for treating cuts and other wounds, eczema, boils, acne, scars, stretch marks, skin ulcers, and inflamed skin. Traditionally, the resin was prepared into various salves and ointments for these purposes, while now the essential oil is used more often.

Mouth

Frankincense is chewed to strengthen teeth and gums and to refresh the mouth. It has antibiotic properties which make it useful for infections of the teeth and gums.

Digestion

Chewing of resin has the secondary benefit of cleansing the digestive system by stimulating bile flow and enzyme secretion and reducing fermentation. A decoction of the resin with cinnamon and cardamom is a traditional formula to relieve stomachache.

Colds

Steam inhalation of the essential oil is an excellent treatment for colds and sinus congestion. Traditionally, the smoke of the smoldering gum was inhaled for treating head colds.

Wounds

Powder of the dried gum is a common ingredient in herbal plasters and pastes used to treat wounds, especially in Chinese medicine. A traditional recipe for an antiseptic wound powder is to mix the powdered resins of frankincense, myrrh, and dried aloe.

Insect Repellant

Burning frankincense in churches had hygienic functions as well as spiritual importance. People of the Middle Ages lived in extremely unsanitary conditions, so the fumigation of churches helped reduce the stench of the unwashed congregants and reduce contagion through atmospheric purification. Burning frankincense also repels mosquitoes and flies.

Memory

The use of frankincense by students for memory and the addition of the resin to coffee, as described above, are based on the resin's memory-enhancing effects. The addition of the resin to coffee is used as a stimulant to treat amnesia.

Rheumatism

While all types of frankincense have anti-rheumatic properties, the Indian frankincense in particular has been utilized by Ayurvedic medicine for this purpose (see Boswellia Serrata and Boswellic Acids below). Use of the essential oil in massage is an excellent treatment for rheumatic and other pains of the muscular system.

Psychological Conditions

Fumigation with frankincense has been used in various cultures to treat a wide range of psychological and emo- tional disorders. In modern aromatherapy, it is used to promote calmness, deeper breathing, and a relaxed state of mind, and is therefore beneficial for depression, anxiety, and mental negativity.

Headaches

Fumigation using the resin is a traditional treatment for headaches. Vaporizing of the essential oil can be used for the same purpose.

Childbirth

In frankincense-gathering regions, gum is burned beside the mother during labor, and the newborn baby is fumigated. Regular fumigation of the baby continues for forty days following the birth. The mother treats herself during this time by squatting over a bowl of the burning gum. This practice assists in the healing of scarring or lacerations, protects the woman from postpartum infections, restores muscle tone, and accelerates recovery.

Decongestant

Frankincense essential oil and fumigation by resin help reduce excessive secretion of mucus.

Respiratory Antiseptic

Frankincense essential oil and resin are used for treating a variety of respiratory problems such as bronchitis and laryngitis. Steam inhalation of the essential oil, combined with other respiratory oils such as eucalyptus, is highly effective. Traditionally, the resin was boiled in goat milk and taken as an antitussive.

Eyes

The resin is a common ingredient in eye washes to treat infections and irritations, as well as a wide variety of ophthalmic diseases. Fumigation with the smoke is considered beneficial to sore or tired eyes.

Cosmetics

Frankincense has countless uses in both modern and traditional cosmetic products. Mixed with beeswax, the resin was once a common treatment for removing darkness and bags under the eyes. Egyptian women use frankincense in various preparations for rejuvenating face masks; it helps improve dry, wrinkled, and aging skin.

Medicinal Uses of Boswellia Serrata

Indian frankincense (Boswellia serrata) has been used extensively in Ayurvedic medicine. Its function is similar to the myrrh-like resin obtained from Commiphora mukul. The Sushruta Samhita and Charak Samhita describe the anti-rheumatic activity of various types of gugguls (oleo gum resins), especially the Boswellia serrata; these texts indicate that these resins have been used medicinally for over a thousand years.

Boswellia Serrata resin is described as having bitter and sweet flavors, with astringent, demulcent, expectorant, antiseptic and anti-inflammatory properties. It is a powerful wound healer and very effective in the treatment of painful joint diseases with inflammation and reduced mobility. It improves blood supply to the affected areas, shrinks inflamed tissue, reduces pain, and enhances repair of local blood vessels damaged by proliferating in- flammation. These effects are attributed to chemical compounds known as boswellic acids, which are now used in contemporary medicine as anti-arthritic and anti-inflammatory pharmacological agents.

Boswellic Acids

The gum resin of Indian frankincense (Boswellia serrata) contains four major pentacyclic triterpenic acids, collectively referred to as boswellic acids. Studies have shown that boswellic acids have an anti-inflammatory action much like conventional non-steroidal anti-inflammatory drugs (NSAIDS). Boswellia inhibits pro-inflam- matory mediators in the body such as leukotrienes. As opposed to NSAIDS, long-term use of Boswellia does not lead to irritation or ulceration of the stomach.

A review of PubMed reports on clinical trials using boswellic acids or resin of Boswellia serrata reveals that these substances have been studied and found highly effective in such conditions as rheumatoid arthritis, osteoarthritis, low back pain, soft tissue rheumatism, myositis, fibrositis, chronic colitis, ulcerative colitis, Crohn's disease, bronchial asthma, and peritumoral brain edemas. Besides its pronounced anti-inflammatory properties, it has been found to have a strong immuno-stimulant activity.

Incensole

There has recently been increased interest in using frankincense essential oil as an anti-cancer agent. The fol- lowing quote is from a personal correspondence with Dr. Ermias Dagne, Addis Ababa, Ethiopia, who is distilling various gum resins for Floracopeia.

"Extracts of Boswellia papyrifera and Boswellia Carteri contain a diter-pene compound called incensole. Incensole is an interesting biologically active compound, reported to have anti-cancer properties. Incensole and other similar diterpene compounds cannot be captured by steam distillation, as they are not highly volatile. About ninety-nine per cent of the resin is thrown out after distillation, but many interesting compounds are present in the residue and hydrosol. Extraction of this residue using food-grade ethanol from organic molasses brings out large proportions of diterpenes, which give the extract a very rich balsamic aroma, with incensole as one of the major components. On the other hand, incensole is only a minor component of the essential oil which is obtained by steam distillation."

Based on this information, we are currently developing a high-incensole ethanol extract of Boswellia papyrifera, which will be used in various formulations.

Myrrh

Origin of the Name

Myrrh is a resin that has a bitter taste; its name is derived from Hebrew murr or maror, meaning bitter.

Origin and Habitat

Myrrh is an oleo gum resin obtained from species of Commiphora trees. There are over fifty species of Commiphora known in Africa, including Commiphora molmol (Somalian myrrh), and Commiphora mada, (Abyssian myrrh). These are small trees of the Burseraceae family, native to the bushland that covers the drier parts of northeastern Africa, Somalia, Arabia, Madagascar, and India. Myrrh is now also found in Ethiopia, Iran, and Thailand.

The major commercial source of myrrh is Commiphora myrrha. However, like frankincense, there are uncertainties about the origin and identity of different types, many of which are not from Commiphoras. Some of the varieties of resin found in the market include Mecca balsam, said to be the myrrh of the Bible; different types of bdellium, including perfumed bdellium, formerly known as East Indian myrrh, African bdellium, opaque bdellium, and Hotai bdellium; and gugul, or Indian bdellium. To further complicate the subject, there are also several varieties of opopanax which are sometimes confused with myrrh, such as Commiphora guidotti, known as sweet myrrh, cassie (Acacia farnesiana), and copal (Copaiba officinalis), an oleoresin which the Catholic church uses in place of myrrh in Central and South America.

Morphology

Myrrh is a thorny tree which grows in thickets to a height of about nine feet, preferring well-drained soil in the sun. The light gray trunk is thick and the main branches are knotted, with smaller branches protruding at a right angle and ending in sharp spines. It has hairless toothed leaves with a large terminal leaflet and two tiny lateral leaflets. Yellow-red flowers grow on stalks in an elongated and branching cluster; they are about five millimeters long and come out just before the rains. The small brown fruits are about one and a half centimeter long, tapering to a pronounced beak. The bark has a silvery sheen and peels in small pieces.

Collection of Resin

Like frankincense, myrrh resin is collected as a thick, strongly aromatic yellow liquid from natural cracks or cuts in the tree bark, which then dries into amber or reddish-brown colored lumps. The tears are found in many sizes, the average being that of a walnut. The surface is rough and powdered, and the pieces are brittle, semitransparent, oily, and often show whitish marks. It is flammable, but less so than frankincense. Adulterations are not easily detected in the powder, so it is better to purchase in bulk so they can be removed.

The oil distilled from myrrh resin is typically thick, pale yellow to orange-brown, with a warm, balsamic, sweet, spicy, and sharp aroma. It has many of the same properties as the resin itself.

Historical and Traditional Uses

Myrrh is one of the oldest medicines in the world. It has been mentioned in Egyptian medical texts since 2,800 BCE, and is one of many herbs mentioned in the Ebers Papyrus, which documents over eight hundred medicinal recipes. The Egyptians consumed large amounts of myrrh, both in temple rituals and embalming; it was also burned in temples of Babylon, Greece, India, Rome and China. It is one of the ingredients of the famous magic-inducing incense, Kyphi, and the ointment Metopian, used for treating infections and wounds. In Chinese medicine, the use of myrrh was recorded as early as 600 CE during the Tang Dynasty, where it was used in a similar manner. Like frankincense, myrrh was an important trade item for more than a thousand years.

Traditionally, myrrh was used for as many diverse purposes as frankincense. It was a primary ingredient in incenses and holy oils used to inspire prayer, deepen meditation, and revitalize the spirit. It was used to fumigate the body to promote cleanliness and stimulate immunity, and continues to have an important role in cosmetics and perfumery. It has also been used to treat cattle and camels, and burned to repel snakes.

Therapeutic Uses

Like frankincense, myrrh resin is a predominant part of the tree's immune system. Many of the therapeutic functions of myrrh are therefore similar to frankincense. A comparison of the two reveals that myrrh is more astringent, antiseptic, disinfectant, bitter, and tonic, while frankincense is more anti-inflammatory, blood vitaliz- ing, and mentally uplifting. The two are often combined. Like frankincense, myrrh has a long history of use for a wide range of conditions, with virtually no toxicity.

The Eclectic physician Dr. Ellingwood describes the therapeutic properties of myrrh as follows: "This agent has always been highly esteemed as a stimulant, although its influence is more of a local than a general character. It exercises the characteristic influence of most of the stimulants upon the excretions and secretions, acting as a di- aphoretic, expectorant, sialagogue, and to a certain extent emmenagogue. As a most active general stimulant in ulcerative, engorged, flabby and atonic conditions of the mucous membranes of the mouth and throat this agent acts promptly. It stimulates the capillary circulation, restores tone and normal secretion and causes the healing of ulcerations. In its influence upon the digestive apparatus myrrh is direct in its action. It quickly increases the power of the digestive function, stimulating the peptic glands to extreme action. It increases the appetite and promotes the absorption and assimilation of nutrition. It is given in atonic dyspepsia in the absence of inflammatory action, especially if there is excessive mucous discharge from the bowels."

Below is a brief list of the most important therapeutic applications of myrrh, which is by no means complete; like frankincense, its uses are so numerous that it can also be described as a panacea.

Mouth and Throat

Myrrh is a specific and highly effective antiseptic astringent for inflammations of the mouth, throat, and gums. It is a common ingredient of herbal tooth-powders and mouthwashes, and is widely used through India and the Middle East for oral and dental problems. The German Commission E has approved myrrh for treating mouth inflammation. Its list of indications includes mouth sores and ulcers, gingivitis, irritation from dentures, sore- ness and looseness of teeth and gums, gum disease, tooth decay, and bad breath. Myrrh is also very effective for infectious and inflammatory conditions of the throat, including strep throat, tonsillitis, and pharyngitis.

For these various symptoms, tincture of myrrh can be diluted and used as a mouthwash and gargle, or applied directly to sores. It is frequently combined with echinacea and/or golden seal for these purposes.

Digestion

In the digestive tract myrrh acts as a stimulant, carminative, tonic, and chologogue. Its bitter principles stimulate the appetite and the flow of digestive juices, improving digestion and absorption. It both relaxes and invigorates the stomach, calming spasms, relieving gas, and combating fatigue associated with weak digestion. Its antibacterial and antifungal powers help reduce candida and other pathogenic factors in the gut. Myrrh has pronounced anti-parasitic properties. By improving digestion myrrh clears toxins from the digestive tract and acts as a general detoxifying and anti-inflammatory remedy, thereby treating the root causes of arthritis, rheumatism, and gout. It can be combined with aloe vera for treatment of both the symptoms and causes of constipation.

Respiratory System

Myrrh is a stimulant, expectorant, and decongestant with antibacterial properties. It is helpful for relieving bronchitis, asthma, and colds. In Ayurvedic terms, it dries kapha (mucous secretions), reduces pitta (antibiotic), and stimulates prana (opens breathing). In Chinese terms, it is a stimulant of Wei Chi (respiratory immune enhancing). It can be a specific remedy for chronic sinusitis. It can be used in carrier oil as a chest rub.

Skin

Myrrh is an astringent antiseptic that is beneficial for acne, rashes, and inflammatory skin problems. The tincture, powder, or essential oil of myrrh can be applied directly to ulcerated sores, wounds, and abrasions. It can be made into salves for treating hemorrhoids and bed sores. For boils it can be taken as a blood cleanser while also being applied externally. It is an excellent addition to the medicine cabinet of those who live in tropical places such as Hawaii, where staph infections can be easily acquired from coral cuts or walking on beaches.

Wounds and Bruising

Myrrh is similar to frankincense in its wound-healing and blood-vitalizing properties, and the two are often combined in liniments.

Antimicrobial and Immune Stimulant

Myrrh is both an antimicrobial agent and a direct stimulant of white blood cell production. It increases resistance to infection, and is one of the most effective of all known disinfectants from the plant kingdom. It is a rejuvenating tonic, and is reputed to enhance of the intellect.

Gynecology

Myrrh acts as an anti-spasmotic circulatory stimulant to the uterus. In this capacity, the resin or tincture is taken for amenorrhea and dysmenorrhea as a purgative of stagnant blood. It helps normalize irregular periods. Myrrh helps promote efficient contractions and relieves pain during childbirth. As an antimicrobial, dilute tincture can be used in vaginal douches. Its internal use should be avoided by pregnant women.

Circulatory System

Myrrh is classified in Chinese medicine as a blood vitalizer with anti-rheumatic and anti-arthritic powers. It is commonly used in liniments and medicated oils for these conditions, as well as general circulatory weakness and stagnation.

Warnings and Contraindications

Myrrh should not be taken orally by women who are pregnant. Oral doses of two to four grams have resulted in kidney irritation and heart rate changes, both of which resolved after individuals stopped taking myrrh. Cases of allergic rashes have been reported from the topical use of myrrh. It may lower blood sugar in some individuals.

Myrrh Abstracts from PubMed

A sampling of studies published on PubMed concerning myrrh derived from different species of Commiphora reveals that the resin reduces cholesterol and triglycerides; that it is a promising non-hepatotoxic anti-helminthic for schistosomiasis; that it is highly effective (100 per cent cure rate) on fascioliasis parasite without remarkable side effects; that its triterpene Myrrhanol A is a more potent anti-inflammatory than hydrocortisone; that it possesses smooth muscle-relaxing properties; that its sesquiterpene fractions had antibacterial and antifungal activity against pathogenic strains of E. coli, Staphylococcus aureus, Pseudomonas aeruginosa and Candida albicans; and that its extract has strong efficacy as an insecticide against the cotton leafworm. In other publications it has been reported that a sesquiterpenoid compound isolated from myrrh is highly effective against drug-resistant tumor cells found in the breast and prostate, without toxicity to healthy cells.

References:

King's American Dispensatory. by Harvey Wickes Felter, M.D., and John Uri Lloyd, Phr. M., Ph. D., 1898.

Furanosesquiterpenes from Commiphora sphaerorocarpa and related adulterants of true myrrh, Fitoterapia, 73, 48-55.Dekebo A, Dagne E, Sterner, O., 2002.

Essential oils of frankincense, myrrh and opopanax. Flavour Fragr. J. 18, 153-156. Baser, KHC., Demirci, B, Dekebo, A, Dagne, E. (2003).

Analgesic effects of myrrh. Nature 379, 29. Dolara, P., Luceri, C., Ghelardini, C., Monserrat, C., Aiolli, S., Luc- eri, F., Lodovici, M., Menichetti, S., Romanelli, M. N. (1996).

Toxcity study in mice of resins of three Commiphora species. SINET: Ethiop. J. Sci. 26, 151-153.Mekonen, Y., Dekebo, A. , Dagne, E. (2003).

Toxicity studies in mice of Commiphora molmol oleo- gum-resin. J. Ethnopharmacol. 76:151-154.Rao, R.M., Khan, Z.A. and Shah, A.H. (2001). Frankincense and Myrrh. Economic Botany 40, 425-433.Tucker A.O. (1986).

Effect of myrrh extract on the liver of normal and bilharzially infected mice an ultrastructural study. Massoud AM, El Ebiary FH, Abd El Salam NF.

Role of circulating Fasciola antigens and IgG4 isotype in assessment of cure from fascioliasis. Hegab MH, Hassan RM.

A safe, effective, herbal antischistosomal therapy derived from myrrh. Sheir Z, Nasr AA, Massoud A, Salama O, Badra GA, El-Shennawy H, Hassan N, Hammad SM.

Preliminary study of therapeutic efficacy of a new fasciolicidal drug derived from Commiphora molmol (myrrh). Massoud A, El Sisi S, Salama O, Massoud A.

New triterpenes, myrrhanol A and myrrhanone A, from guggul-gum resins, and their potent anti-inflammatory effect on adjuvant-induced air-pouch granuloma of mice. Kimura I, Yoshikawa M, Kobayashi S, Sugihara Y, Suzuki M, Oominami H, Murakami T, Matsuda H, Doiphode VV.

Efficacy of the botanical extract (myrrh), chemical insecticides and their combinations on the cotton leafworm, Spodoptera littoralis boisd (Lepidoptera : Noctuidae). Shonouda ML, Farrag RM, Sala

Minor components with smooth muscle relaxing properties from scented myrrh (Commiphora guidotti). Ander- sson M, Bergendorff O, Shan R, Zygmunt P, Sterner O.

Volatile oils of frankincense from Boswellia papyrifera. Bull. Chem. Soc. Ethiop. 13: 93-96.Dekebo, A., Ze- wedu, M., Dagne, E. (1999)

Flavours and fragrances of plant origin, Non-Wood Forest Products, 1, FAO, Rome. Coppen, J.J.W. (1995).

Local anaesthetic, antibacterial and antifungal properties of sesquiterpenes from myrrh. Dolara P, Corte B, Ghe- lardini C, Pugliese AM, Cerbai E, Menichetti S, Lo Nostro

XIII

Essential Oils and the Fifteen Sub-doshas

The objective of this article is twofold. The first is to introduce the fifteen sub-doshas as described by Ayurvedic medicine, which are the anatomical and physiological subdivisions of the three primary doshas of vata, pitta, and kapha. The second is to describe the categories of essential oils that are related to each of the sub-doshas. By describing the functions of each sub-dosha and then correlating essential oils that have direct therapeutic effects on that sub-dosha, we gain an understanding of how the oils affect interrelated systems of organs, channels, and tissues, and therefore know the strengths and weaknesses of using aromatherapy and aromatic plants for different conditions.

Although many oils can be easily correlated with a specific sub-dosha, it is important to remember that essential oils are composed of complex mixtures of molecular compounds, each of which in turn has a wide range of therapeutic actions. It can be accurately stated that every essential oil has multiple therapeutic functions to varying degrees; if these functions are not currently recognized, it is only a matter of time before they are discovered and confirmed by experience and research. Therefore, the assignment of a specific oil to a specific sub-dosha is based on its generally recognized primary therapeutic action, but is not inclusive of every aspect of the oil.

Likewise, each sub-dosha has multiple levels of functions, from the most physical levels of anatomical and physiological activities to the most subtle and innermost activities of the mind and consciousness. The sub-doshas of vata, for example, are closely related to both the breath and the nervous system, but also function at the cognitive level to assimilate sensory information, and at the psychological level to integrate the personality structure and activate the will. Furthermore, these currents of subtle "air" are also said to operate within the realm of spirit, linking consciousness to this present physical incarnation, carrying consciousness into the next incarnation, activating karmic propensities, and other activities that would be considered related to mystical dimensions.

Although aromatic plants have always been ceremonially and ritualistically associated with these subtle realms of consciousness, this article will explore only the most external of the anatomical and physiological sub-doshic activities, with some comments about their mental, emotional and psychological aspects. This article will touch only on the general therapeutic functions of the oils upon the sub-doshas, as the specific pathologies and treatments of each sub-dosha are too numerous to list.

Essential Oils and the Five Vatas

Prana Vata

Prana vata is translated as the "primary air," because of its controlling functions over the other vata sub-doshas as well as the other doshas in general. In this function, prana vata is generally correlated with the nervous system and its control over organ functions.

Prana vata is diffused throughout the head and concentrated within the brain; it could be correlated with brain's neuro-electrical activity that is measured by an EEG. Prana vata governs the sense organs, the mind and consciousness, and assimilates sensory information, emotions, and knowledge.

Prana vata is also called the "forward moving air." In this role it carries food and air into the body; its inward motion governs inhalation and swallowing, while its outward motion is active when sneezing, spitting, and belching.

Prana vata is strengthened and controlled by pranayama, yogic respiratory exercises. In this capacity we can see the interrelationships among breathing, neurological activity and the flow of mental activity and cognitive functions: as breathing is controlled, so are corresponding neurological and mental functions. This aspect of prana vata further clarifies its role as the vital energy that underlies the movement of thoughts and its functions of assimilating mental and emotional sensations into the deeper layers of the psyche and personality structure. Disorders of prana vata are therefore primary causes and symptoms of mental, emotional and psychological suffering.

Prana vata is also one of the major layers of immunological protection. In this role it could be said to be both the neurological aspect of the neuro-hormonal-immunological axis, as well as an aspect of mucus membrane immunology of the sinuses and lungs.

Prana vata and essential oils

Aromatherapy has a direct and intimate relationship with prana vata; this vata is the primary force carrying the neurological effects of aromas via olfaction into the limbic system, into cerebral circulation through the capillary beds of the sinuses, and into the respiratory system. Therefore, all essential oils that are administered through inhalation have a direct effect on prana vata.

Various therapeutic groups of oils can be associated with different levels of prana vata. These are:

1. Oils with respiratory benefits, including mucolytic, expectorant, antitussive, and decongestant functions. These include the conifer oils such as spruce, pine, fir, and juniper; eucalyptus oils; mid to high potency antimicrobial oils such as tea tree, niaouli, oregano, thyme, and tulsi; and resin oils such as frankincense and palo santo.

2. Oils that calm and uplift the shen and rejuvenate vitality through improved sleep and rest (relaxant anxiolytics and nervine tonic anti-depressants). These include lavender, clary sage, palmarosa, geranium, rose, and most other floral oils.

3. Oils that work directly on releasing repressed memories and emotional traumas stored in the subconscious by the limbic system. These include jatamansi, valerian and oils that induce dream activity such as clary sage.

4. Oils that uplift the mind and heart by evoking spiritual moods. These include agarwood, sandalwood, frankincense, palo santo, rose, lotus, and most exotic florals.

5. Oils that enhance cognitive functions in general, specifically concentration, learning and memory, and oils that prevent and reverse neurological degeneration. These include lavender, peppermint, rosemary, and melissa.

One of the most important Ayurvedic treatments that utilizes oils and fragrance for prana vata is shirodhara, a continual cascade of warm scented oil over the head. The warmth and soothing sensation produced by this treatment induces deep relaxation, which could be described as a regression to a prenatal amniotic state. In this state, profound rest and rejuvenation occur within the central nervous system, which in turn produces a multitude of therapeutic benefits. The essential oils that are typically used in this treatment include sandalwood and jatamansi, although shirodhara oils are usually complex mixtures of herbal ingredients.

Udana vata

Udana vata is the "upward moving air" that governs exhalation and speech. Its outer physiological energy is located throughout chest and centered in throat, while its inner subtle function supports memory, strength, effort, and will; it is linked to the powers of discrimination and self-expression.

Udana vata and essential oils

Udana vata is directly related to aromatherapy. As the upward force of exhalation it is benefited by oils that treat the sinuses, lungs and throat. Specifically, all decongestant and mucolytic oils such as eucalypti, conifers, and white sage will directly benefit udana vata when used for inhalation, chest compresses and steam baths. Additionally, the decongestant and mucolytic effects of aromatic herbs taken as hot infusions or decoctions, such as ginger, thyme, oregano, mints, and other common remedies for colds, coughs and respiratory congestion, work on udana vata as the aromatic compounds are exhaled after the first phases of digestion.

Udana vata also functions to support the mind and memory; it might be considered the upward circulatory power of breath that oxygenates the brain. Oils that benefit cognitive functions are therefore also connected to the power of udana vata, especially those that have an upward moving pranic energy such as white sage.

Samana vata

Samana vata is the "equalizing" or "balancing air." Located throughout the small intestine, it could be described as the nerve force of the intestines that governs digestion. It has an inward movement toward center of body, which assists the assimilation of nutrients.

Samana vata and essential oils

The internal use of pure essential oils is contraindicated because of their extremely irritating effects on gastric mucosa. However, the use of aromatic herbs is a primary treatment for this sub-dosha.

Disturbances of samana vata lead to vitiation and accumulation of vata dosha in the form of intestinal gas. Samana vata is treated most effectively with aromatic herbs and spices, whose active principles are essential oils. The numerous genera of the Labiatae family such as Origanum, Ocinum, Mentha, Melissa, Thymus, Rosemarinus, Salvia and Nepeta all help normalize the smooth flow of samana vata. Any type of aromatic tea that contains spices such as ginger, cardamom, cinnamon, coriander, black or long pepper, and fennel, as well as aromatic teas that contain anti-spasmotic functions, such as chamomile and lavender, all work directly on samana vata. A classic example of an aromatic herb that pacifies samana vata by relaxing the nerves is melissa.

Samana vata is also affected by aromatherapy when essential oils are used in conjunction with abdominal massage and abdominal treatments such as ginger compresses.

Vyana vata

Vyana vata is translated as the "diffusing" or "pervasive air." It is centered in the heart, and circulates outward throughout the body. It could be thought of as the vital force of circulation, which governs the blood vessels and gives strength to the musculoskeletal system. Through its action we can express ourselves through movement and activity.

Vyana vata and essential oils

Vyana vata is directly affected during various types of massage. Essential oils used in massage oils, especially those that enhance lymphatic drainage or produce mild rubefacient effects, enhance the benefits for this sub dosha. Camphor, birch, and menthol found in liniments are examples of aromatics that directly affect the superficial levels of vyana vata.

Ayurveda uses numerous complex herbal oils that help oleate the skin, muscles, and joints; this oleation has a supportive effect on vyana vata. These preparations are generally composed of numerous herbal ingredients, including aromatics, which have been cooked slowly for long periods of time in carrier oils such as sesame.

Apana vata

Apana vata is the "downward moving air." It is centered in the colon and governs processes of elimination: urination, defecation, menstruation, sexual functions and childbirth. This sub-dosha is considered the support for the other vatas and exerts a controlling influence on their functions. Regulation and normalization of this vata is a primary goal of traditional therapeutic treatments.

Apana vata and essential oils

Essential oils do not have a direct influence over apana vata when used in typical aromatherapy treatments such as massage, atmospheric diffusing, or steam treatments. Medical aromatherapy uses rectal and vaginal applications of essential oils, which have a direct effect on this sub-dosha. Examples of this would be the use of dilute tea tree for vaginal douching for candida, or lavender oil diluted in a carrier oil as a rectal implant for prostatitis. Calmative, relaxant, and anxiolytic oils can have an indirect effect on apana vata when used for vatagenic conditions such as Irritable Bowel Syndrome. Aromatic herbs are traditionally mixed with laxatives to prevent "griping."

Essential Oils and The Five Pittas

Sadhaka pitta

Sadhaka means the "accomplishing" or "realizing" pitta. Located in the heart and brain, it governs mental energy, digestion of mental impressions and power of discrimination. It could be described as the cellular enzymatic activity within the brain and heart, as pitta is closely connected to agni, the fires of metabolic transformation. At the psychological and emotional level it supports the intellect, intelligence, and ego in accomplishing their goals. This aspect of digestive fire allows the fulfillment of pleasure, wealth, prestige, and spiritual liberation.

Sadhak pitta and essential oils

Sadhaka pitta is directly influenced by oils that have stimulating and tonifying effects on cognitive functions, especially alertness, concentration, and memory. These include melissa, which has documented regenerative effects on acetylcholine receptor sites; gingergrass and other cymbopogon oils, which are nasal decongestants and mental stimulants; lemon-scented oils such as lemongrass (a cymbopogon); citruses in general, especially neroli; and the eucalypti and conifers, which stimulate alertness.

Floral oils and those that create euphoric or aphrodisiac responses, such as jasmine, rose, neroli, ylang ylang and champa, could be considered oils that have a cooling effect upon this sub-dosha, that enhance pleasure by reducing the irritation of pittagenic heat.

Alochaka pitta

Alochaka means "seeing." It is the metabolic fire within the eyes and optic nerve that gives visual perception and allows the eyes to see. Spiritually, it is the clarity within the eyes that reflects spiritual qualities within the being, and the energy that motivates the mind toward clarity and understanding.

Alochaka pitta and essential oils

Essential oils cannot be used directly in or around the eyes. However, all oils that have nasal decongestant effects indirectly benefit this sub-dosha. Many hydrosols (aromatic distillate water) can be highly effective for reducing inflammation or infection (pitta) in the eyes when used as washes. Additionally, many aromatic herbs benefit the eyes through their mucolytic and anti-inflammatory effects on the sinuses.

Pachaka pitta

Pachaka means the "digesting fire." Located in the small intestine, it governs the digestive processes and separates nutrient essence from waste. This sub-dosha of pitta assists in the building of tissues, purification of toxins within food, and regulation of body temperature. It is the basis and support of other pitta sub-doshas and the most important pitta for treatment.

Pachaka pitta and essential oils

Essential oils cannot be ingested directly. However, when deficient, this sub-dosha of pitta is treated with essential oil-containing spices and aromatic herbs. Ayurveda utilizes a large assortment of "pachak" or digestive herbal mixtures for treating low digestive fire, which typically include black pepper, long pepper, ginger, fennel, cardamom, coriander, and various salts. The use of essential oils for culinary purposes has a direct effect on this level of pitta.

Bhrajaka pitta

Bhrajaka means "luster." Located in the skin, this sub-dosha of pitta governs complexion and skin coloration, the digestion of sunlight and the warmth of peripheral circulation. Spiritually, it is that which gives luminosity to the auric field of the body.

Bhrajaka pitta and essential oils

Essential oils play an important role in treating pathologies and maintaining the health of this sub-dosha. If used incorrectly, such as applying caustic or phototoxic essential oils directly to the skin, it is this sub-dosha that responds with inflammatory symptoms of dermatitis. If used correctly, essential oils can be very beneficial for reducing the pitta aggravation of dermal inflammations and infections.

Essential oils have been used for millennia for treating this sub-dosha, in the form of ointments, unguents, washes, sprays, and other cosmetic applications. Many oils are gentle yet potent anti-inflammatories, such as lavender, frankincense, rose, geranium, and chamomile, which are cosmetic ingredients with ancient histories. Many of these oils also have strong wound healing, scar tissue-resolving, and skin rejuvenating powers; the helichrysum oils are one the best known examples.

In addition to essential oils, hydrosols and fatty oils can also be included in treatments of bhrajaka pitta. Abhyanga, oleation with massage, has been the primary treatment for maintaining the health, integrity, and immunological strength of this sub-dosha.

Ranjaka pitta

Ranjaka means "color." Located in the liver, spleen, stomach and small intestine, this sub-dosha is responsible for giving color to the blood, feces and urine. It could be regarded as the cycle of bile, from the degradation of red blood cells in the spleen to the secretion of bile into the small intestine and into the feces.

Ranjaka pitta and essential oils

Essential oils do not have a direct effect on ranjaka pitta.

Essential Oils and The Five Kaphas

Tarpaka kapha

Tarpaka means "contentment." Located in the brain, heart and cerebro-spinal fluid, this sub-dosha of kapha provides nutrition, strength, and lubrication to the nerves. Emotionally, it provides emotional calmness and stability; it also plays an important role in supporting the functions of memory. Spiritually, it gives inner happiness and joy, mental contentment and bliss. It is regenerated through meditation.

Tarpaka kapha and essential oils

Aromatherapy has a direct effect on tarpaka kapha. As one of the sub-doshas of the brain, there is a direct link between aromatherapy, the limbic system and consciousness. The oils most directly beneficial for this sub-dosha include those that enhance memory and concentration, including melissa, rosemary and citruses; nurturing floral relaxants that pacify overstimulation of vata and pitta such as lavender, clary sage, chamomile, geranium, and rose; the sacred scents that evoke contemplative and devotional moods such as agarwood, sandalwood, rose, lotus, palo santo, and frankincense; and oils that release traumatic memories stored by the limbic system, such as valerian and jatamansi.

As with treatment of prana vata, the profound relaxation induced by the warm oil treatment of shirodhara has a profound effect on this sub-dosha.

Bodhaka kapha

Bodhaka means "perceiving." Located in the mouth, tongue and saliva, this sub-dosha of kapha governs the sense of taste and initiates the first stages of digestion.

Bodhaka kapha and essential oils

Aromatherapy is directly related to bodhaka kapha. Loss of taste is frequently secondary to the loss of smell. In some cases, depending on the cause, loss of smell can be restored using aromatherapy. Additionally, essential oil-containing spices and aromatic herbs act directly on this kapha when consumed with food or as teas.

Kledaka kapha

Kledaka means "moistening." Located in the stomach, this sub-dosha of kapha is the alkaline secretions of the mucous membranes of the GI tract. It governs the liquefaction of food during first stages of digestion, controls the watery elements of the digestive process, protects against the acidic properties of pitta, and helps the movement of nutrients from the GI tract to the tissues.

Kledaka kapha and essential oils

Decreased digestive fire leads to increase of kapha, both locally and systemically; when there is an accumulation and excess of kledaka kapha in the GI tract, aromatic spices and herbs are a primary treatment. The essential oil-containing aromatic medicines used in these cases have digestive properties including carminative, mucolytic, stomachic, anti-spasmotic, and cholegogic. This list includes the entire range of culinary herbs and spices: cardamom, fennel; ginger, black pepper, long pepper, basil, bay leaves, coriander, cumin, dill, hyssop, marjoram, oregano, thyme, peppermint, rosemary, sage, and many others.

Sleshaka kapha

Sleshaka means "lubrication." Located in the joints, this kapha produces the synovial fluids. It functions to hold joints together and to give ease of movement. It provides strength and stability in movement.

Sleshaka kapha and essential oils

This sub-dosha of kapha is directly benefited when essential oils are used in the treatment of musculoskeletal injuries and arthritis; a wide range of anti-inflammatory oils are beneficial for these conditions. Frankincense, helichrysum, jatamansi, and sweet birch are primary oils for reducing inflammation (pitta) that affect the joints, while fatty carrier oils such as sesame, coconut, almond and numerous others give hydration to sleshaka kapha.

Avalambaka kapha

Avalambaka means "supporting." Located in the heart and lungs, this sub-dosha is the storehouse of kapha that controls the other kapha sub-doshas; it is the primary kapha. At the physical level it is the phlegm produced by the lungs; it also has an affinity with the blood plasma. Emotionally, this sub-dosha is responsible for the creation of emotional attachments.

Avalamaka kapha and essential oils

This sub-dosha is directly affected by respiratory essential oils that have expectorant, decongestant, and antitussive effects, including eucalypti, conifers, angelica, white sage, and frankincense. The use of these oils is especially beneficial when used in steam inhalations and compresses. The routine use of these oils in atmospheric diffusing is an excellent way of protecting the immunological integrity of this sub-dosha from mold and contagion of colds and flus.

XIV

Medicines For The Earth
The Eco-Physiology of Plants

Introduction

We are entering a period in history when human health will be seriously challenged. If the destructive trends of rapid global warming, accelerating loss of biodiversity, widespread pollution and degradation of ecosystems, deepening poverty, malnutrition, and political instability are not reversed, all forms of medicine will become increasingly ineffective, unaffordable, and unavailable. For large populations in many parts of the world, this future has already arrived.

The causes of these conditions are numerous, complex, pervasive, and seemingly overwhelming. There is, however, one solution that has the potential to unify humanity in worldwide healing—the plants.

Plants are the foundation of civilization and culture. They created the biosphere of the earth's surface, and they regulate its functions. Plants are the ultimate source of all health and prosperity; they feed us, give us clothing and shelter, provide fuel, fiber, and countless other necessities. Every breath we breathe is the breath of plants, which supports all life. Plants are the origin of medicine.

When healing an illness, there is often relatively little that doctors and patients can do to directly produce optimum functioning of human physiology. Plants, however, provide the biochemical and nutritional compounds that assist the body's internal ecology and promote its innate homeostasis and equilibrium. Phytonutrients nourish the organs, support the tissues, and enhance immunity, while the medicinal constituents of botanical species detoxify metabolic waste and xenobiotics (harmful foreign substances). No synthetic pharmaceutical drug can perform these functions.

Similarly, there is relatively little that people can do to reverse global warming, to stabilize disturbed weather patterns, or to detoxify environmental contamination. But plants do all of these things. They cool the planet, help regulate the seasons, recharge groundwater, restore soil fertility and stop erosion, regenerate the ozone layer, bind atmospheric carbon dioxide, and purify the toxins we put everywhere. Plants perform the same crucial functions in the outer environment as they do in the inner environment of the body.

This article, along with "The People's Pharmacy" and "The Pharmacy of Flowers," outlines a broad vision of plants as humanity's primary resource for solving the complex and potentially devastating challenges we face. The article begins with a brief overview of how plants created and sustain the biosphere, followed by an exploration of the parallels between human and plant physiology, and comparisons between disease processes in the human body and planetary ecosystems. Finally, it outlines some of the ways plants are being used for healing the environment, and how these functions are similar to healing mechanisms in the human body.

Plant physiology and planetary evolution

The life-supporting elements that we often take for granted are the result of unimaginably long cycles of evolutionary processes. It can accurately be said that plants created, and continue to create, the world we live in. Recognizing our dependency on the eco-functions performed by plants increases our sensitivity to the conditions of the environment, and encourages us to protect and restore the natural world.

From the perspective of plant eco-physiology, four events are of major significance in the long biological history of the earth. The first is the appearance of single-celled photosynthetic organisms in the primordial ocean about three billion years ago. This pre-plant photosynthesis brought about three planetary changes: the radiant energy of sunlight began to be converted into chemical energy, which became the nutritive foundation for all subsequent life forms; atmospheric oxygen increased, which allowed the evolution of more complex organisms and life forms; and atmospheric oxygen was converted to ozone, which provided protection from solar ultraviolet radiation and allowed migration of life onto land.

The second evolutionary step was the migration of multi-celled organisms, the precursors of modern plants and animals, onto land about 450 million years ago. By 400 million years ago, early vascular plants were radiating across the land.

The third important development was the evolution of plant roots. By 375 million years ago, root structures penetrated almost a meter into the soil. This development brought about major changes in the soil and atmosphere; between 400 and 350 million years ago a 10-fold decrease in atmospheric carbon dioxide occurred, as a result of plant respiration and microbial activity in the root systems.

The fourth evolutionary step occurred around 100 million years ago, with the appearance of flowering plants. This relatively sudden development brought about a rapid expansion of biodiversity, culminating in human beings, as new forms of life evolved in symbiotic relationships with the plant realm.

Similarities Between Plant and Human Anatomy and Physiology

Plants and humans share numerous anatomical and physiological characteristics; we are actually more similar than different. Understanding these remarkable parallels gives us a greater appreciation for the kinship that exists between the plant and human realms, which in turn is the basis of reverence for nature and respectful coexistence with biodiversity.

The similarities between plants and humans can be simplified into three categories: basic life needs, anatomical and physiological characteristics, and subtle functions.

Basic life needs

The basic needs of plants and people are the same. Plants and people share the fundamental biological cycle of birth (germination), growing to maturity, reproduction, aging and decline, and death. Plants and people both need nutrients in order to grow and thrive, water to moisten the tissues and facilitate metabolic processes, air for respiration, and environmental and seasonal conditions conducive to life. Plants and people both need defense mechanisms to protect themselves from the elements and from other organisms; both suffer from diseases, viral and bacterial infections, and parasitic infestations.

Anatomical and physiological characteristics

There are numerous parallels between the anatomical structures and physiological functions of plants and people. Plants have outer cells that function similarly to skin. Just as human skin is lubricated and protected from the external elements by oily secretions of the sebaceous glands, the aerial surfaces of plants secrete wax produced from fatty acid precursors for waterproofing and immunity. Human bodies are shaped and supported by bony skeletons, while plants have their own connective tissues and skeletal structures; the growth and development of plant cells and organs rely on a skeleton comprised principally of microtubules and microfilaments. The blood vessels and capillaries of the human body can be compared to the xylem (wood) of plants, which is a complex vascular tissue containing water-conducting cells; the blood and lymph correlate with the various fluids that flow through the channels of the plants. The human alimentary canal is comparable to the roots, which draw nourishment into the outer tissues and cells of the plant. Humans and plants both have reproductive systems; human sperm and ova can be compared to the pollen-producing stamens and ovary-containing pistils.

Like humans, plants have complex immune systems. Plants produce purely mechanical defenses, such as spines and thorns. Chemically, they secrete essential oils and oleoresins, which function as immunological compounds to discourage herbivores, stimulate healing of wounds, and protect from insect and fungal pathogens. Plants react to pathogens and diseases by producing certain antibacterial compounds; phytoalexins are probably the most studied of these defensive compounds. These immune responses can be compared to various responses of the human immune system, such as the activation of lymphocytes.

Plant metabolic functions are governed by hormones, as are human functions. Gibberellins are one group of hormones that control growth and a wide variety of other plant developmental processes.

Plants have detoxification mechanisms that work to break down xenobiotics; many of these mechanisms are similar to how the human body deals with toxic compounds. Both plants and humans require certain nutrients and enzymes to efficiently remove toxins and to protect themselves from stress. For example, glutathione plays an important role in various physiological processes of both plants and humans, functioning primarily as an antioxidant.

Like humans, plants suffer oxidative stress and free radical damage when exposed to xenobiotic compounds, and produce antioxidants in response. Pollutant tolerance in plants is determined by many of the same physiological mechanisms as in humans. In general, there are more similarities between the metabolic pathways of plants and humans than there are differences.

The bodies of plants, like the bodies of humans, support complex microbial ecosystems. From the root tips to the tips of the highest leaves, plants provide a diverse habitat for a wide range of microorganisms. Just as the skin and mucous membranes of the human body are the biogeography for various colonies, each zone of a plant has its own cohort of microorganisms. Both the human and the plant body set the stage for its microbial inhabitants, and in turn, the microbes establish a range of varied relationships with their partners, ranging from relatively inconsequential transient visits, to symbiotic functions, to pathogenic attacks.

Subtle functions

There are other fascinating parallels between plants and humans that are more in the realm of subtle energetic physiology than purely biochemical or anatomical functions. Plants, like humans, have circadian rhythms. There is accumulating evidence that plants have multiple circadian clocks both in different tissues and, quite probably, within individual cells. Plant growth, like the growth of the human body, is guided by gravity. Gravitropism, the ability of plant organs to use gravity, has been recognized for over two centuries. Like the human body, plants develop symmetry of form; like the human body, these processes arise in embryogenesis. Plants communicate, both with other plants and with other forms of life. The primary signaling mechanism for this is semiochemicals. These secreted compounds act as attractants and repellants of beneficial or destructive insects, and allow plants to inform other plants of events such as insect attacks and infestation. Studies have also demonstrated that plant growth is stimulated by certain kinds of music and inhibited by others, indicating some level of sensory awareness and sentience.

Parallels Between Human Illness and Biospheric Disorders

One of the most remarkable aspects of traditional Asian medical systems is the practice of diagnosing and treating illness as disequilibrium of nature's elements within the microcosm of the human body. Ayurvedic and Chinese medicine describes physiological activity using imagery of external elemental forces as they manifest within the individual organs and tissues, such as heart fire, heat in the liver, wind disturbing the nervous system, spleen dampness, and lung dryness.

The implications of this philosophy are both profound and scientifically accurate. It reveals that we are inseparable from nature; that we are composed of nature's elements; that these elements are continuously circulating into, through, and out of the body; that the body functions according to the same laws as the planetary biosphere; and that nature's intelligence strives to restore equilibrium within the body. This knowledge of biological interrelatedness and interdependency, which is the basis of many yogic and contemplative practices, is urgently relevant for our modern world.

Traditional Asian medicine is fundamentally a system of "eco-physiology," which applies the principles of terrestrial ecology to the functioning of the human body. These universal principles are not only applicable to the human body, however - they can also be used to help diagnose and treat disturbances of the biosphere. Using the holistic humoral and energetic models of traditional Asian medical systems, a number of correlations can be made between disorders within the human body (microcosm) and the biospheric functions of the earth (macrocosm). Exploring these similarities is a kind of "macro-thinking" that helps develop awareness of the unity of body and nature; it is also important for clinical success, since illnesses are inseparable from the outer elements and increasingly related to environmental factors. Without this holistic perspective, it is difficult to identify and remove the root causes of illnesses, and natural medicine loses much of its depth and power. The relevance of this knowledge to plant eco-physiology is that both the internal and external aspects of diseases are corrected by the physiological functions of plants.

The most critical disease process occurring at the planetary level is global warming. From an eco-physiological viewpoint, global warming is a fever of the earth. Global warming in turn creates the conditions for epidemics of infectious febrile diseases. Drought and desertification, two increasingly severe manifestations of global warming, can be compared to dehydration and yin deficiency syndromes, which are also generated by chronic heat conditions. In the same way that botanical medicines provide a wide range of anti-inflammatory, antibiotic, and demulcent compounds, plants are the key to reversing global warming and desertification through their oxygen-generating, carbon-dioxide-binding, water-recycling, and environmental-cooling functions.

Water pollution in the outer environment can be closely correlated with various forms of fluid toxicity that affect tissues. Water pollution, water stagnation, and the generation of pathogens are closely linked, as when dams create overgrowth of malarial mosquitoes or microbial pathogens. In the body, fluid stagnation, fluid toxicity, and the overgrowth of pathogens are also closely related, as when chronic phlegmatic congestion breeds opportunistic viral and bacterial infections of the respiratory tract, or lymphatic stagnation leads to inflammatory skin conditions. Botanical medicines effectively treat fluid stagnation and toxicity syndromes; plants are also the primary agents for remediation of water pollution and purification of microbial ecologies.

Contamination of the soil can be compared to contamination of the bodily terrain, especially the digestive tract. Loss of topsoil and depletion of soil fertility leads to malnutrition, which is depletion of the body's tissues. Depletion, toxicity, and genetic modification of the plant kingdom are a fundamental cause of nutritional disorders; both can be linked through the concept of the "earth" element in Chinese and Ayurvedic medicine. Plants are the primary source of nutrients for the body and its tissues, and they are also the primary agents of soil regeneration and the most important way of preventing erosion of topsoil.

A wide range of further parallels can be made between human and biospheric physiology. Erratic weather patterns generated by global warming can be described as disordered biorhythms. "Dead zones" in the ocean created by agricultural toxins can be compared to necrotic tissues of the body. Fascinating comparisons can be made between various diseases, such as cancer and AIDS, and their corresponding manifestations in the biosphere. More examples will be explored below.

Parallels between antibiotic and pesticide use

Another important series of correlations can be made between the effects of antibiotics and the effects of pesticides. Philosophically, antibiotics and pesticides both reflect the nature-dominating paradigm of modern Western culture. Medically and ecologically, both practices are unsustainable. Economically, their use is driven primarily by corporate profit motive.

The relevance of this information to plant eco-physiology is that plants are the solution to the worldwide problems caused by antibiotics and pesticides in both the micro and macro ecosystems. Medically, the phytonutrients, alkaloid compounds, immune-enhancing polysaccharides, and essential oils of botanical species will become increasingly important as microbial virulence increases and antibiotics lose their effectiveness. Ecologically, the revival of biodynamic and organic gardening methods will replace toxic agricultural chemicals as pesticide and herbicide resistance increases.

Antibiotics and pesticides both target unwanted organisms. Both destroy the complex healthy microbial communities in the various terrains where they are used; antibiotics destroy healthy intestinal, mucous membrane, and skin flora, while pesticides destroy the microbial communities in the soil and natural predators such as beneficial insects and birds. Both approaches lead to increased resistance and virulence in bacteria, insect pests, and invasive weeds. The use of both is followed by a rebound effect: overgrowth of candida and other opportunistic infections after antibiotic use, and flourishing of insect pests after the effects of spraying have worn off. Antibiotics weaken immunity, while pesticides and herbicides decrease soil fertility and plant resistance. Increased pathogenic virulence and resistance combined with weakened host immunity leads to susceptibility to re-infection after antibiotic use, and susceptibility of plants to opportunistic diseases after pesticide use. Antibiotics lead to accumulation of toxicity within tissues and organs after repeated use, while pesticides and herbicides lead to accumulation of chemical toxicity in soil, water, and air.

Parallels between organic gardening and natural medicine

On the other hand, parallels and analogies can be made between the non-toxic methods used in organic gardening and farming, and the principles of natural healing. Both activities are based on the eco-physiology of plants, whether in the garden or in the body.

Building healthy soil by promoting microbial communities through composting has an obvious correlation with improving digestive function by building healthy intestinal bacterial ecology. Insects attack plants with poor immunity, just as bacteria opportunistically attack weaknesses in immune defenses. Increasing biodiversity, such as integrated pest management and companion planting, increases plant resistance; in a similar way, botanical medicine and integrated therapies strive to strengthen the body through the use of a broader spectrum of nutrients and healthy stimuli. Using aromatic plants to repel insects in gardens is similar to the use of essential oils to treat bacterial and viral infections. Increasing the availability of oxygen and nutrients to tissues by increasing circulation is similar to supplying nutrients to plants through proper aeration of soil. Providing good drainage of water in the garden is comparable to improving fluid metabolism and removing congestion.

Phytoremediation: Using plants to heal the environment

Phytoremediation is the removal and degradation of contamination in soils and groundwater by plants. It utilizes a variety of plant physiological functions, including direct uptake of toxins, metabolism of those toxins into less toxic or nontoxic compounds, and degradative processes of bacteria and fungi within plant root systems. These processes, which are capable of removing low to moderate levels of environmental pollution, can be correlated with similar functions in the human body, which also degrade and eliminate xenobiotics and metabolic waste.

There are many advantages of using phytoremediation over conventional remediation methods: it is less expensive, it can be applied to a wide range of toxic metals and radionuclides, it is minimally disruptive to the environment, it is solar powered and energy efficient, it requires little maintenance, and it is aesthetically pleasing. There are thousands of phytoremediation projects in different stages of research and development around the world.

A wide range of environmental toxins can be remediated using plants. Phytoremediation is being used to clean up metals, pesticides, solvents, explosives, crude oil, polyaromatic hydrocarbons, and landfills. Hybrid poplar and Eastern cottonwood remove chlorinated solvents in ground water. Petroleum and its hydrocarbons can be removed from soil and ground water using alfalfa, poplar and juniper, fescue grass, crabgrass, and clover. Polyaromatic hydrocarbons are remediated with ryegrass and mulberry trees. Heavy metals can be removed from soil using poplar and pine trees, chaparral, various grasses, and castor plants. Radionuclides can be removed from ground water with sunflowers and water hyacinth, and from the soil with mustards and cabbage. Explosives such as TNT can be removed from groundwater with duckweed and parrot feather grass. Nitrates can be remediated with cottonwood and poplar trees. Various water plants, including hyacinths, are being used in municipal sewage treatment.

In the last five years it has become clear that while phytoremediation has significant benefits in certain applications, its widespread commercial use is limited by the natural processes of plant physiology: plants degrade toxins slowly, large areas are needed for planting, many plants cannot be grown in the soils and climates where they are needed, and much remains unknown about the field in general. The scientific community involved in this research is now exploring genetic modification of plant physiology as a way of enhancing their remediating powers.

Some improvements in plant remediation capacity using genetic modification have been reported, such as using bacterial genes to help plants degrade mercury more efficiently. By inserting mammalian genes to express cytochrome P450 liver enzymes, plants have been modified to enhance their degradation of trichloroethylene, a ubiquitous toxic solvent used in dry cleaning.

It is ironic that scientific advances intended for human betterment are the original source of the chemical, biological, and nuclear waste that now needs remediating. It seems likely that the well-intentioned efforts to improve plant functions with genetic modification, like much of modern allopathic medicine, may yield symptomatic benefits while worsening the overall health of the biosphere. Holistic medicine, on the other hand, addresses the causative factors of illness and works to eliminate them. The obvious solutions to widespread contamination of the earth is to first stop manufacturing and using toxic substances (detoxifying the patient from addictions), converting to nontoxic plant-based alternatives (creating a healthy lifestyle), and enhancing phytoremediation capacities by restoring ecosystems to their original biodiversity (restoring systemic immunity and homeostasis).

The Eco-Physiology of Phytoremediation

Phytoremediation can be categorized into six basic plant functions: phytodegradation, phytoextraction, rhizofiltration, rhizodegradation, phytostabilization, and phytovolatilization. These functions are clear examples of the eco-physiology of plants and its practical applications for environmental remediation. Several comparisons can be made between these plant processes and human metabolic functions.

Phytodegradation

Phytodegradation, also known as phytotransformation, is the breakdown of contaminants by metabolic processes within the plant, or the breakdown of contaminants external to the plant through the effect of compounds produced by the plants. Plants degrade contaminants through enzymatic pathways, and the metabolites are incorporated into new plant material. Phytodegradation processes are effective on organic pollutants including petroleum byproducts, pesticides like DDT, and explosives like TNT.

The processes of phytodegradation can be compared to detoxification processes in the human body, especially those occurring in the liver, such as the cytochrome enzymatic pathways.

Phytoextraction

Phytoextraction is the use of plants to absorb toxic metals from the soil into the harvestable parts of the roots, stems, and leaves. "Hyper-accumulators" absorb unusually large amounts of metals in comparison to other plants. One or a combination of these plants is selected and planted at a particular site based on the type of metals present. After the plants have been allowed to grow for some time, they are harvested and either incinerated or composted to recycle the metals. Approximately 400 species of hyper-accumulators exist, including representatives of many families from herbs to perennial shrubs and trees.

Unlike phytodegradation, the plant does not destroy or use the material, but simply stores it; as it absorbs more from the soil, concentrations of the substance within the plant can become extraordinarily high. For example, the tree Sebertia acuminata absorbs so much nickel that it bleeds a blue-green latex when cut, caused by the oxidized nickel. Metals such as nickel, zinc, and copper are preferred by a majority of the hyper-accumulating plants; others absorb radioactive strontium, cesium, and uranium.

Phytoextraction can be used to pull contamination from water deep in the earth. Because trees are the largest plants in the world, they are able to take up more contaminants than other plants. Poplar trees are being used to extract the widely used solvent trichloroethylene from soil and water. Ninety-five percent of the solvent can be removed from groundwater by simply planting the trees and letting them grow, and about ninety percent of the solvent is degraded into harmless compounds. Through this function of hydraulic pumping, trees also prevent the spread of contaminated water to other areas.

Phytoextraction of toxins by plants is analogous to the accumulation of toxins within the organs and tissues, especially the liver.

Rhizofiltration

Rhizofiltration is similar to phytoextraction, but the plants are used primarily to address contaminated ground water rather than soil. The rhizosphere (the area surrounding roots of plants) contains 10 to 100 times the amounts of bacteria in unplanted soil; organic compounds degrade faster in this microbe-rich area. As the roots become saturated with contaminants, they are harvested. For example, sunflowers were used successfully to remove radioactive contaminants from pond water in a test at Chernobyl.

Rhizodegradation

Rhizodegradation is the breakdown of contaminants in the soil through microbial activity in the root zone (rhizosphere). Certain microorganisms can digest organic substances such as fuels or solvents that are hazardous to humans and break them down into harmless products. Plants release sugars, alcohols, and acids from their roots, which provide nutrition for the microorganisms and enhance their activity. Biodegradation is also aided by plants loosening the soil and transporting water to the area.

The degradative and detoxifying effects of the microbial rhizosphere during rhizofiltration and rhizodegradation are similar to functions performed by beneficial intestinal flora in humans. Using the rhizosphere of plants to enhance bacterial activity in soil is comparable to using probiotic supplementation to remove pathogens such as candida and their toxins.

Phytostabilization

Phytostabilization is the use of plants to immobilize contaminants through absorption and accumulation by roots, adsorption onto roots, or precipitation within the rhizosphere. This process does not remove the toxins from the soil, but reduces their mobility, prevents their migration into groundwater and air, and decreases their entry into the food chain. Poplar trees, for example, can transpire between 50 and 300 gallons of water per day out of the ground. The water consumption by the plants decreases the tendency of surface contaminants to move towards ground water and into drinking water.

A simple parallel can be drawn between the use of plants to stabilize toxins, and the body's natural mechanism of encapsulation to prevent the spread of various toxins into the blood and tissues.

Phytovolatilization

Phytovolatilization is the uptake and transpiration of a contaminant by a plant, with release of the contaminant into the atmosphere. Phytovolatilization occurs as trees and other plants take up water and the organic contaminants. Some of these contaminants can pass through the plants to the leaves and evaporate, or volatilize, into the atmosphere.

The leaves of plants are like lungs: both are responsible for respiration and volatilization of waste gases.

Medicinal Plants Used in Eco-Restoration

Several plants with important nutritional and medicinal properties are being utilized in ecological restoration and environmental remediation. These species represent a unique category of phytoremeditation and plant eco-physiology: plants which benefit the environment while simultaneously providing food and medicine. Four examples are kelp, neem trees, vetiver grass, and sea buckthorn.

Kelp

There are several species of kelp, which are among the fastest growing plants in the world. Kelp produces more oxygen and binds more carbon than any other sea plant; studies suggest that if the original kelp beds of the world's oceans were replanted (one percent of the ocean's surface), they could stabilize atmospheric carbon dioxide levels, the primary greenhouse gas associated with global warming. Kelp forests purify coastal ecosystems and provide habitat for fish populations. Kelp, like other sea vegetables, is a highly nutritious food and medicine, used specifically for supporting thyroid functions.

Neem (Azadirachta Indica)

Neem trees are an excellent example of an agro-forestry crop that remediates environmental pollution while providing a wide range of medicinal and agricultural products. The trees improve soil fertility, rehabilitate degraded wastelands, control soil erosion, and prevent floods; they can withstand extreme heat and high levels of water pollution. Because they provide numerous items of commerce, neem plantations are a panacea for economically depressed areas. The United Nations has declared neem the "tree of the 21st century" because of the many solutions to global problems that it offers.

In India, neem is considered the "village pharmacy." Every part of the tree provides a variety of medicinal substances for a vast range of symptoms. Neem leaves are a potent hepatoprotective agent; they are effective against parasitic infections, have significant anti-ulcer activity, and are strongly anti-inflammatory. Neem bark is used as a bitter tonic with antibacterial properties; it is effective against a number of skin conditions, including eczema, burns, herpes, scabies, dermatitis, warts, and dandruff. The fatty oil expressed from the seed has a long history of use as a nontoxic spermicidal contraceptive; it also reduces uterine inflammation. A large number of herbal pharmaceuticals, cosmetics, and body care products are now based on neem products.

One of the best examples of plant eco-physiology is nontoxic pesticides produced from neem leaves. Neem-based pest control products, like herbal antibiotics, have broad-spectrum modes of action that are not only effective against pests, but also safer, less persistent in the environment, and less prone to pest resistance than synthetic pesticides.

The bioactivity of neem has been extensively evaluated and is well established. It is the only plant from which effective and eco-friendly bio-pesticides are commercially manufactured. Neem pesticides are used in India on crops like cotton, vegetables, fruit trees, coffee, tea, rice and spices. The EPA has approved the use of neem products on food crops in the US, as well as for ornamental and landscape plants. Neem products are being used in commercial-scale crop management in Canada. Neem-based pesticides are expected to capture 10 percent of the global pesticide market by the next decade.

Another application of neem's eco-physiology is nontoxic fertilizer. Neem leaves, like many herbal medicines with bitter principles, have dual functions:

Indian farmers have traditionally used neem as a fertilizer which also acts as a pest repellent. Neem leaves simultaneously enrich the soil and protect plant roots from nematodes, ants, fungi, and harmful bacteria.

Vetiver (Vetiver Zizanioides)

Vetiver is a grass with important phytoremediating functions. Because of its deep and complex root system, it is one of the best grass species for preventing soil erosion. In China, vetiver is being planted on a large scale for pollution control and phytostabilization of mine tailings. Vetiver roots also function as a highly efficient filter for rainwater, slowing down runoff, controlling floods, and recharging ground water. In places where vetiver is planted the soil moisture and groundwater are significantly improved: water levels in wells are higher, springs do not dry up, and small streams run longer into the dry season.

Vetiver roots absorb and transform agricultural toxins. The grass thrives in polluted water and improves both the quantity and quality of the water. It is effective in removing agricultural phosphates and nitrogen, and it mitigates environmental problems resulting from toxic minerals. There is evidence that vetiver can remove pesticides as well.

Vetiver improves soil fertility and crop production. When used as an amendment, it improves soil nutrients and increases crop yields. Vetiver protects orchards by reducing the temperature in and above the soil and increasing air moisture

Vetiver is easy to establish, is inexpensive, and needs minimum maintenance. It thrives in a wide range of ecosystems and different soil types, can withstand serious drought and long-term water logging, is more tolerant of hot and cold than the other grasses, and is not seriously affected by pests or diseases. It promotes the growth of other plants and helps restore vegetation.

Vetiver is now being grown for environmental purposes in over 100 countries. It provides a number of important items to households and farms, such as fragrant sleeping mats, thatching for roofs, mulch, and animal feed. Vetiver is the source of an aromatic oil used in perfumery, incense, and medicine.

Sea Buckthorn (Hippophae rhamnoides)

Sea buckthorn is a shrub that has been used for numerous purposes for at least 1,200 years. It is mentioned in Tibetan medical classics from the sixth century. Until the 1980s its use was limited to Tibet and Mongolia; now it is cultivated for a variety of purposes in China and other places.

The eco-physiology of sea buckthorn has valuable environmental applications, while simultaneously providing numerous medicines, foods, and cosmetics. The primary ecological benefits of the shrub, like vetiver grass, are based on its complex and deep root system, which provides excellent soil-binding properties, erosion control, and stabilization of mountainsides.

Conclusion

The overall health of society is determined more by its nutritional, hygienic, and environmental status than by the sophistication of its medical systems. If medicine does not address these underlying levels of wellbeing and illness, it is not holistic. Physicians and healthcare practitioners of all disciplines have a responsibility to support planetary ecological health by identifying the causes of diseases and educating patients about how to remove those causes. As this holistic consciousness increases throughout society, the recognition of plants as agents of both medical and ecological healing will also increase; this awareness, in turn, has the potential to dramatically change the destructive priorities of modern society and lead to the creation of sustainable, prosperous, and peaceful plant-based cultures. In my opinion, this is the most important goal of medical practice today.

XV

Keynote Speech to the National Ayurvedic Medical Association

April 20th, 2012, Bellevue, WA

Welcome to everyone, from near and far.

It is a great honor to be invited to give the opening presentation at this conference. It is especially an honor considering that I don't have a formal education in this medical tradition, not even a two year certificate training from a program here in the US.

My education in Ayurveda has happened in other ways. I have approached the subject more as a traveling ethnobotanist, a journalist, photographer and filmmaker, a person interested in cultures and history, someone who loves plants and the natural environment, a clinician with a background originally in Traditional Chinese Medicine, a writer and poet occasionally visited by the muses, and a normal bewildered human who tries to make sense of the world through the unique paradoxes of our species. These experiences have perhaps given me a perspective on Ayurveda that I might not have gained by academic study, although I have undertaken those studies at various times, but found that I can't remember anything for very long.

Therefore, my relationship with Ayurveda has been one of avoiding discussion about the subjects where I am weak, meaning most of what is taught in schools and practiced in clinics, and focusing instead on its more universal themes. This has proven to be a fairly effective strategy, and apparently, sufficient for those who invited me here. Thank you for that.

There is certainly no deficiency of universal themes in Ayurveda. I will give you some examples that have special meaning to me.

Have you seen the cardamom forests of Kerala? They are a vision of grandeur, and a living testament to the question of whether people can live in harmony with nature or not. Towering trees dropping delicate flowers onto the cardamom's broad leaves; the air filled with melodic bird songs and the sound of streams and waterfalls; the smell of rich fertile earth. It has been this way for centuries, as the massive trunks covered with vines of black pepper show. It was this way when

Columbus set off, hoping to find Port Kochin, where those mountains meet the sea. For those in search of precious spices, this was the promised land; for me, it was proof that enchantment still lives somewhere in the world.

Have you visited the sandalwood forests, where the last of this precious species grows? It is a unique experience to savor the exquisite aroma that emerges from under the bark, and to know that this fragrance is not only the essence of the tree's heart and all the years it has known, but also the essence and heart of so much of what Ayurveda means, with its sattvic beneficence that nourishes our body and mind with something that pharmaceutical medicine never will.

Have you ever walked in fields of tulsi where old women from the last agrarian generation labor all day in sweltering humidity, twice as strong as modernized young men half their age, and still radiant with toothless smiles? It is easy to understand why this herb is sacred when you hold it to your face, its freshly harvested aroma mingling with the scent of the steaming fields, its green foliage against the backdrop of white egrets taking wing, an herbal treasure destined to become medicine for everyone, protection for homes, and an offering that brings joy to the deities.

Have you seen the fields of roses that spread out below Savitri's temple that rises above Lake Pushkar in Rajasthan, blossoming in the approaching light of dawn as if the goddess of radiance were sending waves of perfumed color across the desert to announce her arrival?

I could go on in this vein for a long time, because it is so rich, and pleasurable, so full of sensual healing imagery. It is about the beauty of the plants, and our ancient relationship with them. It is about how botanical intelligence can preserve what is left of the natural world, and regenerate the rest before it is too late. It is about how people can have work, and livelihoods that have been the backbone of societies for millennia. It is about how men, women and children have seen the presence of divinity within trees and flowers and herbs, and have brought that vision to life with myth and legend and poetry and ritual. It is about how those myths and rituals have bonded people safely together into communities that have endured and endured for longer than the imagination, generation after generation further back than memory, as if out of time.

It is about the profundity of what was seen, comprehended and taught by those we call the Seers and Sages of this lineage, and the aspiration that arises when sacred knowledge enters consciousness that others may also see and comprehend this profundity, and what that means to us at a time when our ignorance is so deep that we are destroying that which gives us life.

That is what this presentation is about. It's not about Ayurveda as a medical system, although that is part of it. It's about what Ayurveda tells us about life, and nature, and the presence of the sun and moon within us, and how that knowledge might help us see that light inside each other. It's not about the herbal market, or clinical therapies, although that is part of it. It's about our universal human needs, and how this ancient tradition advises us how we may fulfill those needs, and our hopes and dreams and creative impulses and spiritual aspirations, and leave the world a better place than we arrived when we dissolve into formless peace.

I like to set challenges for myself. Or, to be more honest, I need to have challenges given to me, otherwise I tend to become comfortably tamasic. When I was invited to give this talk, the only thing required was the title. That was the easy part. Six months later, I can report that I have spent a lot of time wondering what the title actually means, and how to discuss it in a meaningful way.

Ayurveda: The Global Language.

The first impression one might get from this title is that I have some insights into how our healing methods might become a global phenomenon: how Ayurveda might become our national health care system, how it might help our politicians develop wisdom and compassion, how the life-giving practices of Vedic agriculture might change the minds of those who modify the genetics of our foods, how nontoxic plant medicines might replace the overuse of pharmaceutical drugs, how meditation and yoga might be taught in schools, how healthy food might wean children off Ritalin, how hospitals might offer pancha karma. It is a hopeful vision.

When we think this way, are we not thinking of ways to bring more Ayurveda into the world? That has been my dream. Many people are dreaming of this, and working toward these goals and accomplishing some of them, and to these people we owe our collective presence here, just as our presence affirms that we have all contributed to accomplishing something very significant for Ayurveda.

This is one of the meanings of the title: how we can continue to bring Ayurveda into the world. And there are so many ways, and so many pleasures of contemplating them, and of seeing how they can solve so many problems, and even more, seeing them do so. Even with so little time, we will cover some of these topics, and hopefully leave here with a broader understanding of the potential ways that we can further integrate Ayurveda into our complex, troubled, brilliant, distracted, modern culture.

Ayurveda: The Global Language

There is another interpretation of this title, one that is in a way the opposite of bringing Ayurveda more fully into the world. It is that of bringing the world into Ayurveda.

This interpretation is based on understanding that Ayurveda, for all its deep and encompassing and urgently relevant universal themes, is limited in many ways. Many of its most important contributions to the world are still bound by history and culture and geography, by language, by mythology and religion, by politics and legal issues, and by the reality that it depends on valuable plants that are being overharvested. It is based on the reality that for all its benefits, proven both empirically and scientifically, traditional cultures want to be modern. It is based on the reality that while many are working tirelessly to create a more holistic medical system in the West, political powers are driving economic forces in the opposite direction, and that healthcare in this country is increasingly dominated by the will of insurance company executives, who are not motivated by compassion, and Ayurveda, therefore, is not on the agenda.

This pragmatic understanding of Ayurveda's limitations can help us avoid the temptation to think in utopian terms, which I for one am prone to do. The world that is rapidly unfolding now confronts us with an undeniable truth: the forces of nature are more powerful than our utopian visions. Therefore, we must strive to increase Ayurveda through the channels that we know, which are primarily education, clinical practice, lifestyle counseling and herbal medicine, but we must also begin to question what is Ayurveda's higher purpose, in our individual lives, in society, and for the earth?

If, because of increasing financial limitations, its medical applications can only play a limited role as an out of pocket luxury, a few herbal products or a rare healing retreat, what else does Ayurveda offer our suffering world? It is, after all, the noble "science of life," that has brought healing to kings and peasants, humans and animals, soil and water, so we should not feel timid about asking this.

So what does it mean, specifically, to bring the world into Ayurveda?

First, it means to recognize that the world is already full of Ayurveda, in countless forms that are not called by that name, yet are in fact of the same essence, meaning, application and result.

Second, it means to embody Ayurveda, in ways that go far beyond simply knowing its methods and talking its talk. Ayurveda, after all, is the living energetic and elemental reality of our physiology, and therefore accessible to everyone regardless of national, cultural, racial, ethnic or religious habits of the ahamkar.

What specifically does it mean that the world is already full of Ayurveda? I will give you a preview of my thoughts.

Ayurveda becomes limited to geography and culture when we use the term "Ayurvedic herbs." When we say "herbs used according to the Ayurvedic system of knowledge," it becomes a global language, that holds within its pharmacopeia not just the plants of the Indian subcontinent, but all plants of the earth. How many of those plants are understood in terms of their rasa, virya and vipak and their relationship to the doshas and dhatus? Only a tiny fraction I am sure. Suddenly, there is vast potential to bring the world into Ayurveda, and that is only at the botanical level.

I think of my good friend Arjun Das, a teacher and practitioner of Ayurveda and jyotish who lives in Bela Horizonte, Brazil. Those of you who know Arjun may feel the same way about him that I do, which is that he is a young Rishi with a deep organic understanding of Ayurvedic wisdom. His work is exemplary of how Ayurveda can function as a community building force. He has his clinic, which is full; he has a full team of interns; he has students all over the country, and travels extensively to teach; he has started and maintains several large herb cultivating projects; he has opened an Ayurvedic hospital to serve the poor; he takes people to India for intensive trainings with traditional Vaidyes. These are all ways that he has brought Ayurveda into the world.

But Arjun is also bringing the world into Ayurveda. Because of the corruption and political control by pharmaceutical companies, it is almost impossible for him to import Ayurvedic medicines from India. Instead, he has undertaken the immense project of classifying Brazil's botanical pharmacopeia into the language of Ayurveda. Now, after many years of working with his students to gather, organize and preserve the ethnobotanical knowledge from the traditional people of the mountains and jungles, Arjun has created a system of using Brazilian herbs according to Ayurvedic diagnostic and therapeutic principles.

This was done exactly as the Ayurvedic writer Todaramalla advised, and the same way Ayurvedic herbal knowledge grew in India, by learning about the plants from the tribal people of the forest and translating those functions into the cosmology of gunas, mahabhutas, doshas and dhatus. What Arjun has accomplished now offers a clear road for other practitioners of Ayurveda to travel as this medical system spreads into this botanically wealthy country. Even more importantly, as time passes, more and more people will take up this challenge, and the vast pharmacopeia of Ayurveda will become even larger.

Now we come to an important exercise, that of defining Ayurveda outside of the cultural, geographical, botanical, religious, linguistic, and political appearances that currently define it, and most people's understanding of it. By doing so, we may find that Ayurveda is already far more widespread, powerful and influential than we realize, and that its wisdom and insights can be expressed in many more forms than we imagine.

We might ask, for example, what other sciences qualify as a "science of life."

Monsanto knows a lot about the science of life.

Pharmaceutical companies know a lot about the science of life.

Oil companies know a lot about the science of life.

Nuclear engineers know a lot about the science of life.

Astrophysics knows a lot about the science of life.

And in truth, people working in these fields know far more than the Rishis and traditional Vaidyes did, about the genetic intelligence within plants, and microbes and molecules and their effects, about geology and energy systems, about the atomic world, about the formation of stars and world systems.

But what is wrong with this picture? If these are indeed sciences of life, why are they threatening the future of life on earth?

And so we come to an important criteria that defines Ayurveda as a global language. It is not the "science of life" as much as the "science of living," because science and its understanding of life has far surpassed Ayurveda's antiquated understanding. It is, to be precise, the "science of nurturing and protecting life," which clearly distinguishes its purpose from modern science and its dubious and often dangerous applications.

With this definition, we can now see that those who care for the soil and the seeds by practicing organic agriculture are part of Ayurveda's global presence and future, while companies such as Monsanto are a threat to everything that Ayurveda represents. We can see that medicines for attacking and subduing microbes are destined to be overcome by them, and out of the failures of drug resistance will come the realization that Ayurveda's guidance to live a symbiotic life, not an antibiotic life, is indeed wise.

We can see that our addiction to oil and uranium is nothing more than willful ignorance of how to utilize cleaner forms of energy, and that those who are developing those forms are in fact accomplishing the same results of balancing agni and removing toxic pitta and ama, but from the channels and tissues of the earth instead of the human body. We can see that those who probe the farthest reaches of the universe and tell us of their visions are likewise modern Sages, who inspire the same wonder and awe that the cosmology of the ancients pointed to, while those who apply this knowledge to military purposes threaten what Ayurveda seeks to protect.

So we have now brought into Ayurveda the entire range of global botanical biodiversity, as well as other great fields of inquiry and practice that are also expressing the knowledge and wisdom that Ayurveda propounds: that of ecological agriculture, that of nontoxic and humane developments in medicine, that of alternative renewable energy, and that of sciences that genuinely deepen our respect and love of nature. And there are many more.

Suddenly, Ayurveda appears to be much larger and more relevant to the world than an ancient medical system that is dependent on herbs from India and based on Sanskrit texts and mysterious cosmological principles. Instead, it begins to look like the best qualities of the human psyche that are expressing themselves in every place and culture in response to the damage caused by our darker, more selfish and generally unconscious drives, at a time when the outcome may indeed determine our continued biological existence.

From this perspective, the goals of Ayurveda appear to be in solidarity with many social, environmental, economic and spiritual movements that do not even know the name Ayurveda, but share its vision and aspirations.

And in the center of this global drama, grow the plants.

Plants are the original communities. Plant communities are the foundation of all other communities, starting with pollinators and culminating with human civilization. If we want to bring Ayurveda into the world and the world into Ayurveda, we must understand our relationship to plants and the role they play in creating and sustaining communities.

Ayurveda has taught me some very important things about our relationship with plants.

The plants are what hold the formless awareness of Purush in Prakruti's embrace.

How is this? Without plants we would have no nourishment to provide a home for our mind, and without plants there would be no nourishment for the womb to bring forth another generation of life. Therefore, in order for Purush to incarnate into Prakruti, it must cross the bridge from energy to matter, and then be nourished so that it can remain there.

Plants are the bridge that connects the external five elements with the internal seven dhatus; across this bridge flows the solar agni, with one end starting in the sun and the other radiating from the light of our eyes. On one end is photosynthesis, on the other is human metabolism, its mirror image.

Ayurveda taught me about agni. I contemplated the sensations of agni in my body, and came to understand that its warmth was sunlight harvested by the plants.

Here is something else Ayurveda has taught me about our relationship with plants.

Almost the entire food chain comes from flowering plants: grains, fruits, vegetables, legumes…these are all flowers. In order to reproduce, flowers offer nectar to pollinators.

Ayurveda tells us that sweet is the only flavor that directly builds and nourishes the dhatus. We know that the end result of metabolism is ojas, which is described as nectar gathered from the seven dhatus, a nectar that has the taste of honey, but we also know that the end result of metabolism is glucose.

Therefore, just as there is a bridge that carries agni from the sun into our bodies, there is also a bridge that carries sweetness from the flowers into the final vipak of our tissues.

Ayurveda has taught me that we are solar powered beings that live on nectar.

In spite of our sophisticated neurological capacity, our place in the web of existence is only as secure as the vanishing pollinators that weave together the flowering foods we depend on, and the bridge of light they create between the sun and the warmth of our hearts.

Knowing this, we are faced with a biological imperative: to preserve the botanical ground of our being and the foundation of biodiversity that it supports, or to leave this planet to other more adaptable life forms. This simple truth has the power to change all of our social, economic, and political priorities. This simple truth is inherent in the fundamental teachings of Ayurveda, because without stability and health of the biosphere there can be no balance of the doshas, dhatus and malas within the individual, there can be no happiness of mind and clarity of sense organs, and there can be no fulfillment of the four aims of life. Therefore, Ayurveda also leads us to the same global biological imperative.

I will share something else that I have learned from Ayurveda about the plants and our relationship with them and their role in healing communities.

Just as the external elements of earth, water, fire and air enter and circulate through the channels of space inside the human body, so it is in the bodies of plants. Just as these elements are carried by currents of prana in the human body, so it is in the bodies of plants. Just as the human body is influenced by the sun and moon, the seasons, the health of the soil and water and air, so it is with the bodies of plants.

In botany and agriculture, the term eco-physiology is used to describe the effects of the environment and ecological factors on the physiology of plants. By studying eco-physiology from the perspective of Ayurveda, we learn that the rasa, virya, and vipak of plants are composed of the five elements that they have extracted from the landscape, which are infused with the twenty qualities of the sun and moon that awaken and bring forth the pranic intelligence latent in their seeds.

The language of Ayurveda is therefore the language of eco-physiology, because it describes the effects, the imbalances and the treatment of the outer environmental elements as they circulate through the human body.

The obvious implication is that we can learn to see the gunas of the sun and moon such as hot and cold, and the presence of the five elements within the microcosm of the body, and learn how to regulate them. The less obvious implication is the converse: that we can see the vitiation of the doshas, the congestion of the channels, the disturbances of agni, the accumulation of ama, the depletion of ojas, and every other Ayurvedic description of eco-physiological disturbance, in the biosphere of the earth.

It would be an interesting use of our time to unpack all these fascinating parallels and describe them in Ayurvedic medical language. What is global warming in the language of the doshas? What is acidification of the oceans in the language of ama? What is loss of topsoil and the destruction of the ozone layer in the language of the dhatus? What is the proliferation of jellyfish, an oil spill in the Gulf of Mexico, the radioactive plumes of Fukushima, and the way that cities appear like tumors from space?

But there is something more important to discover, because in the center of this drama grow the plants.

And all they want to do is harvest sunlight with their green hands, and transform it into nutrients, and with those nutrients grow and thrive and reproduce, in the process making food and air for all other living beings.

But that is not all they do. Just as they regulate the inner ecology of the human body, so do they regulate the outer ecology of the earth. Just as they purify the inner elements of the body, so do they purify the outer soil, water, sunlight and air. Just as they nourish the body, so do they nourish the biosphere.

Plants, therefore, are not only the bridge between Prakruti and Purush, and the source of sweetness that becomes the nectar that fills our cells, but also the agents of nature's self organizing intelligence, the prana that regulates the elements, in both the outer and the inner biospheres.

So we come to another way to understand Ayurveda as a global language, and that is all the diverse ways that we could be using plants to purify and regenerate our planetary home, from community and school gardens to reforestation to massive projects of phytoremediation.

If we define Ayurveda this way, we might think of Paul Stamets, and his pioneering work with mycoremediation, the use of fungi for healing and detoxifying the earth. Besides his numerous successful projects detoxifying oil spills and contamination from military waste, he has proposed a "nuclear forest" in response to the disaster at Fukushima, designed to hold, stabilize and gradually decompose the ongoing radioactive contamination, using the prana, tejas and ojas of the trees, shrubs, roots and fungi.

To me, this is an example of the visionary macrothinking of Ayurvedic eco-physiology; it also appears to be suspiciously like a Rishi might think. It is inspiring to me to know that there are such Rishis among us, who not only understand the secrets of nature but are also motivated by compassion to apply them to helping the world. It is even more inspiring to realize that Paul is only one person in an entire generation of bioneers who are seeing, developing and implementing such systems of biological healing. I imagine that it will not be much longer before our community of practitioners and other such communities of scientists, philosophers and practitioners begin to collaborate and cross pollinate to create novel and innovative ways to "nurture and protect life."

Ayurveda grew from an agrarian culture and an environment of rich biodiversity. It has both a special responsibility and a special ability to protect and restore that culture and the environment, and this is why its larger aims and goals are in solidarity with other sciences and practices such as phytoremediation, organic agriculture and renewable energy. In my opinion, this solidarity makes our efforts to bring Ayurveda into the world a heroic undertaking, because it is part of a larger struggle to establish Dharmic consciousness and livelihoods in the face of deeply entrenched resistance from profoundly corrupted wealth and power.

And so let's examine some of the heroic ways that Ayurveda is being brought more into the world, starting with the plants, because the presence of plants is one of many ways that communities are healed. Just as there are many vaidyas who have left India to carry the message and methods of Ayurveda to other countries, there are hundreds of botanical species that have also emigrated from their homeland.

Here is an example of a person who does not come from a background of Ayurveda, but is playing a central role in bringing this form of medicine to the US. Richo Cech is one of the world's experts on cultivation of medicinal plants for their seeds. I asked him "How many species of traditional Ayurvedic herbs do you sell, and how many people are planting them?" He told me that he grows and sells over one hundred species, and that those seeds go to many thousands of people every year.

I imagine that most people would probably think of the spread of Ayurveda as more students graduating from more schools and opening more clinics to serve more communities, and this is true. But let's not forget the original healers that cause the metabolic transformations within the body, and remember that the spread of Ayurveda is also more people planting more seeds and harvesting more flowers and roots and sharing more teas and herbal remedies from the garden with more friends and families.

If I were asked to share a great moment in the transmission of Ayurveda to this country and how it helps communities, I would tell you that two summers ago my friend William Siff got some tulsi seeds from Richo and grew huge amounts of it on his farm in the Berkshires of Massachusetts for his clinic, and that one beautiful afternoon I found myself in a big circle of students sitting around a gigantic bed of this fine sattvic herb in all its aromatic flowering glory, with Hillary Garivaltis leading everyone in pranayam.

Here was the essence of Ayurveda as a global language: people from all over the country, an herb from India that is now well established in the US as a medicinal and cash crop, and the transmission of Ayurvedic and yogic teachings.

What stands out in my memory about that sacred moment was that this plant had brought together not only a community of people who shared a love for Ayurveda and its botanical treasures and their uses, but also a community of creatures that felt the same way. As we humans sat inhaling the uplifting fragrance of tulsi's purifying breath, we were surrounded by butterflies, honeybees, and a multitude of other grateful beings enjoying her nectar.

But it was not only the creatures and the students that were grateful for the presence of the holy basil that fine summer day, but also a large extended family of those who had been touched by its presence throughout the region.

The reason I was there at William's Goldthread Farm was because of an important educational program that he launched four years ago, called Farm to Pharmacy. I took the liberty to invite myself to be his co-teacher, because I believe that what William is doing is extremely important for the local community, for society, for the earth, and for plant based medical lineages, and I wanted to support him.

I also had a selfish motivation, which was that I wanted to get closer to the medicinal plants, and do healthy work like digging roots of ashwaghanda and trimming the tulsi flowers. This desire to get closer to the herbs is what draws most students to this program, and the place where most of them first encounter Ayurvedic teachings. Working directly with medicinal plants on a farm or in the garden is one of the most important and one of the most neglected aspects of hands on training in Ayurveda, and it is one of the most exciting ways that we can promote the spread of this medical tradition into our communities.

When we begin caretaking and harvesting the plants that are used in treatments and formulas, we are replanting the roots of Ayurveda. In the process of doing so, the plants begin weaving communities together and supporting community health in ways that do not happen simply from clinical practice.

Ayurveda came from an agrarian culture and is dependent on plants, and in order to preserve its clinical practices and increase its presence in the world, it must have strong roots in the soil of local farms and gardens. Therefore, I believe that American students growing tulsi and ashwaghanda and numerous other species represent a revolutionary development in the growth of Ayurveda, and the first step in establishing the truly holistic vision of Ayurveda in our culture.

At the Goldthread Farm and Apothecary we can see many ways that these medicinal plants are weaving together threads of new communities and supporting community health.

The first way is the direct contact with the plants. By planting their seeds, caring for them as they grow, harvesting them and making medicines from them, students gain a much deeper level of knowledge than using products from plants they have never met. If you have never dug the deep roots of ashwaghanda from rich soil, you cannot fully appreciate its pranic power; if you have never trimmed the flowers of tulsi or spread its fragrant leaves on drying racks you cannot fully know its beneficence.

The second way is that this pranic vitality immediately benefits the patients who use these plants. We know that through the good work of several Ayurvedic companies that we now have access to high quality and high potency organic herbs from India. This is extremely important not only for the land where they are grown and the people who cultivate these crops, but also because it allows us here in the US to utilize many important species that do not grow here. However, there is nothing that compares to the healing power of fresh herbs grown and harvested locally.

The herbs that are grown and harvested at Goldthread Farm go into three primary channels. The first is that William uses them in his clinical practice.

The second is that they are sold in the apothecary. In both cases we see that the community benefits from the presence of fresh and vital plants, and each patient in turn experiences superior results with Ayurvedic medicine.

The third channel of distribution is completely unique, and represents an innovative model of healthcare for communities. This is what William calls Community Supported Medicine, or CSM. This is based on the well known model of Community Supported Agriculture, except that instead of buying shares for produce, people buy shares for a seasonal box of herbal teas, tinctures, syrups and other remedies for the home and family. I personally believe that this simple system is the future of nontoxic and affordable healthcare in our country; I imagine that the collective sharing of herbs in this way is probably very similar to the way ancient Ayurveda was practiced at the local village level for millennia.

The herbs from the farm are reaching the community in other ways as well. One is that other local farmers are now getting involved in growing many of these species, to help supply William's clinic and apothecary. Another is that the nurses of the local school district are now using herbal teas from the farm for simple complaints instead of routine medications. Giving children tulsi and peppermint teas for stomach aches may seem to us like natural thing to do, but getting such herbs into a public school is not a small or simple thing in this backward country; therefore, I consider this form of community outreach a particularly spectacular and revolutionary development in the history of Ayurveda in the West.

I took the time to describe this one person and one farm because it is an innovative and critically needed model of community healthcare that brings fresh and potent Ayurvedic medicinal plants and the knowledge of their use into local communities. However, this is only one of many such projects that are beginning to sprout around the country, and one of our explicitly stated goals in doing the Farm to Pharmacy series is to train people to become community herbalists who can duplicate this model in their own neighborhoods.

We can take the previous example of only tulsi and multiply it by one hundred times the number of other species Richo tells us that he sells, then multiply that by several thousand times the number of people he sells to, then multiply that times an unknown number of other seed companies and nurseries that sell an increasing range of Ayurvedic medicinal plants and all their clients and all the farms that are starting to discover the Farm to Pharmacy model and we can start to see a wonderful vision of Ayurveda spreading across the US in the form of countless gardens filled with flowers, herbaceous plants, medicinal roots, trees and shrubs, culinary spices, and vines. And as they go, each of these herbal emissaries carry their prana, tejas and ojas into the communities that they have invaded, and soon the knowledge of their use for healing will follow, as it did when Ayurveda was first born.

That knowledge will follow, because those medicines have often been planted by Ayurvedic practitioners, or a practitioner will soon discover them in their vicinity, because Ayurvedic practitioners, like weeds and invasive species, are springing up everywhere.

I could not go far in the development of this little talk without wondering "How far and how wide has the name of Ayurveda travelled in modern time, and what forms is it taking as it spreads?"

Using the powerful mudra called "point and click," I paid homage to the greatest Rishi of our time, the omniscient Google-ji. The results were quite interesting. Instantaneously, I discovered a directory listing Ayurvedic practitioners in 37 states in the US, including BAM's, medical doctors and chiropractors. I could easily imagine Ayurveda taking root in urban centers such as Los Angeles and New York City, but I couldn't help but wonder how it is being received in Kansas and Oklahoma.

An instant later I found another directory with 9307 practitioners in 762 cities around the world, from Burma to Israel to Mexico to Scotland.

The next directory had even more countries with Ayurveda, and I became curious about how this great river of healing is faring in a place such as South Africa; I discovered 8 practitioners in that directory alone, all looking very healthy and happy and offering wonderful services.

Several countries appear to have become home to numerous clinics and practitioners, such as Russia and Brazil. In Europe there is a counterpart to NAMA, appropriately named Eurama. We can also add the local counterpart here in Washington, WAMA, and we have a formidable lineup: NAMA, WAMA and Eurama as antidotes to ama and as alternatives to the AMA.

Within a few minutes, this little exercise began to stimulate my cravings for massage and shirodhara, especially when I started perusing the tantalizing websites of gorgeous five star hotels that have adopted our healing methods. Would I go to the Maldives first, would it be Tyrol in the Alps, a mineral spring in Bulgaria, or a private reserve with treatment rooms in caves in Africa?

It is impossible to know what percentage of practitioners in these diverse places have planted gardens with seeds from India in their communities, but we do know that wherever Ayurveda is practiced, it creates a community of people who start to become healthier and happier, and that every practitioner is to varying degrees a catalyst of positive change in that community.

Ayurveda is growing, developing and unfolding in concert with other disciplines that are not part of its history, and it is also growing with lineages that have always been closely entwined with it. We do not need to spend time on the profound impact that Vedanta has made on Western culture for over a hundred years, or the impact more recently of yoga and kirtan, as the effects of these can be easily seen in almost every progressive community.

Instead, I would like to mention agnihotra, a practice that seems to have an intriguing magical effect on harmonizing the mahabhutas of the environment in a way to heals disturbances within communities, balances the weather patterns, increases fertility of the soil and crop yields, reduces environmental toxicity, plant diseases and pests, and produces numerous other benefits. This ancient but recently revived practice appears to me to be a perfect interface between Ayurveda and agriculture, environmental restoration and rejuvenation, and communities.

Here are some brief quotes, by people who are benefitting from this practice, which is both universal in its essence and also unique to Vedic culture. All of these people are living in Columbia, where much healing is needed; I am sure these statements would make the Rishis happy.

Jose Magmud, a doctor of Homeopathy says: "As soon as we did agnihotra on the farm, it started raining. It had not rained for two years!"

Miguel Zapata, a medical doctor says: "I introduced "this practice" to some friends who had a farm in Casemare close to Boyacá. This area was affected by the paramilitaries who would steal cows and kill people. After they started with the practice, these paramilitaries became their friends and protected them."

Olga Martinez says: "I work with children who have learning disabilities and autism. At the beginning, when I start working with a group, some children hit the walls, bite, scream, jump and are very difficult to manage. Then I started doing agnihotra for ten minutes. After that the children become quiet and ready to work. It calms down the children right away."

Martha Restrepo, says: "We have been practicing for four years. Little by little, peace and tranquility pervaded the house and the problems with the teenagers and neighbors disappeared. After some time, the whole block was peaceful. We have learned to be tolerant and teach how to be tolerant by example. Many people like my children because they have an aura of peace around them. Before, we tried to grow some plants and we couldn't. Now, we have an avocado tree and a small jungle in the front and backyard of our house. It was very dangerous to walk out at nighttime for anybody. Now it is safe. It is truly a miracle because usually these things are very difficult to change."

A farmer from a cold region with bad soil reports that his production of fruits almost doubled. He says:

"We produced enough veggies and fruits for the whole town. It was incredible! We received First Prize for Ecological Production. The following year, we again received the First Prize."

He goes on to say that after starting agnihotra, the flow of water from their source increased by seven times.

This farmer concludes: "My wife and I realized that it was all due to Homa, which transformed the soil into this spectacular land! We didn't realize how powerful Homa was until now."

All of these marvelous results happened from this: placing some grains of rice into the flame of a burning piece of ghee-saturated cow dung in a small copper pyramid and reciting a mantra while facing the rising or setting sun.

I have always associated the healing benefits of agnihotra with the Ayurvedic writings of Charak. Charak is said to be a Rishi, although historians think that he might have actually been several people. I think of him as a Seer who predicted global warming, 2,500 years ago, by seeing cause and effect and holistic interrelationships between people and nature.

In one of the verses of his Samhita, dedicated to infectious diseases, he makes the astute observation that epidemics are caused by corruption within the government. He elaborates, by telling us that when leaders become corrupt, they deceive the people and lead them from a life of Dharma into wrong livelihoods. When people leave the life of Dharma, they neglect the sacred activities, and instead, their unhealthy activities generate heat toxins, which accumulate in the atmosphere. The accumulation of heat toxins from non-Dharmic living in turn causes displeasure in the realms of the sky devas, and the rains do not come on time. First there is drought, then there are floods, and the seeds cannot grow. Food becomes scarce, people become weak, and they are susceptible to epidemics. This happens when people follow corrupt leaders.

Agnihotra, therefore, appears to be a revived non-sectarian form of an ancient Vedic practice that helps people reestablish a Dharmic relationship with the elements and pranic intelligence of the sun, the plants, the soil, water and air, and in the process make the devas of nature happy again, resulting in peaceful conditions and increased abundance. This is the foundation for achieving the stated goals of Ayurveda: balance of the doshas, dhatus and malas, happiness and clarity of the senses and mind, and the attainment of the four aims of life.

Now we come to another interpretation of the title of this talk. What makes Ayurveda a global language is its power to communicate directly with everyone, to communicate what is most important and needed by people everywhere, and to communicate at levels that transcend all our external superficial differences.

Relatively few people know the concepts or the language of Vaidyas, but everyone everywhere understands the language of soothing touch. Not everyone cares about vata or pitta, but everyone is afraid of pain and inflammation. Not everyone can relate to kitchari and ghee, but everyone knows the difference between hunger and satiation. Everyone suffers when the body is filled with sensations of toxicity and exhaustion, and everyone feels joy and happiness when those sensations are replaced with purification and rejuvenation.

Every human being needs Ayurveda. Every man, woman and child, no matter what their age, no matter what the status of their health, can benefit from Ayurveda. This cannot be said of modern pharmaceutical medicine.

For twenty years I have been saying that you can read the entire Physician's Desk Reference and not find a single drug that provides nutrition to the body, or that detoxifies the organs and tissues. It is a simple truth that cannot be denied. I have said that pharmaceutical medicine has an important role in the world, but its great limitation is the inability to increase vitality and immunity with nutrition or to cleanse and purify, and therefore it cannot address the fundamental root causes of almost all sicknesses, at a time when the quality of the food chain is increasingly compromised and the toxicity of the world is rapidly rising.

What Ayurveda offers, therefore, is fundamentally more important, more necessary and more effective at raising the levels of health in communities than pharmaceutical medicine ever will. As we know, if there was even a little bit more Ayurveda in the world, there would be far less need for pharmaceuticals.

This is because Ayurveda is fundamentally nutritive and purifying, and humanity needs nutrition and detoxification more than it needs more drugs to cope with the symptoms of nutritional deficiency and excess toxicity.

Ayurveda is nutritive and purifying for the body, for the emotions, and for the mind. If it is nutritive and purifying for the individual, it will have nutritive and purifying effects for the family. As families receive nutrition and purification of body, emotions and mind, communities will become healthier.

All practitioners of Ayurveda increase the health of the community with their work. Each massage, each shirodhara, each person who improves their diet, each person who gradually cleanses and rejuvenates their body and mind, contributes to the community becoming healthier.

Ayurveda, therefore, is a perfect venue, medium and opportunity for community outreach, community development, and healing of communities on a larger scale than working with individuals one to one in the clinic.

When I started writing this section, I realized that a significant percentage of people in this audience are doing something with Ayurveda outside of their clinical practices that represents this broader level of community healing, especially if we use the wider definition of Ayurveda's shared goals with other Dharmic, social, economic, and ecological movements.

Without looking far, I thought of those that I have some direct personal contact and interaction with that are worthy of special mention.

I am most impressed with the agricultural work of both Banyan Botanicals and Organic India, and the huge impact that both of these companies have made at the ground level to give healthy employment and bring poverty alleviation to large numbers of people through the production of high quality organic crops. But these are only two that I have some connection to, and I imagine that every company present in the vendor hall deserves honorable mention in this way.

Likewise, every school represented here is having a positive influence on local communities, not only through education but also through their clinical facilities, their gardens and other special projects.

On a personal level, I am big admirer of the heroic work of Sarita Shrestha, and a supporter of her hospital, Devi Ma Kunja, that serves impoverished women in Kathmandu. I think Sarita's journeys to the remote villages of Nepal to provide Ayurvedic medicines to thousands of people at a time is as inspiring an example of community outreach as we could find.

I am also an admirer of the work of Niika Quistgard and Rasa Ayurveda Center in Kerala, specifically for her project that educates women of the local villages so that they continue to know and use their own local herbs at a time when traditions are being quickly forgotten.

I am also a great admirer of Ruth Hartung, who has created dynamic and powerful affiliations between her 7 Centers Yoga Arts and foundations such as Gardens for Humanity. This partnership has resulted in a renaissance of locally produced organic foods and medicinal plants, celebrated every year as the Sedona Spring Planting Festival. Among Ruth's many accomplishments is integrating the local botanical species of the desert into her Ayurvedic teachings, creating a new form of truly grassroots healthcare.

There are so many people worthy of recognition for their great contributions and accomplishments, that it would have been easy to use this entire lecture to simply mention them. I will conclude this brief list with an observation of what I have seen in my travels and know from my involvement with not only these projects, but many others.

Almost every one of these endeavors is underfunded. Almost everything that everyone is accomplishing in these diverse approaches to Ayurvedic community outreach, whether it is clinical, educational, environmental, ethnobotanical, or whatever, is being done as seva, out of compassion and a desire to help humanity. Everyone is working with very little economic support from the sectors of society that should be contributing the most. In this sense, Ayurveda also shares solidarity with the other global Dharmic struggles, that are almost universally operating with shrinking budgets as increasing amounts of the world's wealth continues to concentrate in the hands of fewer and fewer.

Now we have come to the last section of this talk, not because there is a deficiency of universal themes or heroic stories, but because I will soon wear out my welcome.

We have seen some ways that the world can be brought into Ayurveda, and how its purposes are in alignment with many other important global movements. We have seen some examples of people who are bringing Ayurveda into the world, and hopefully from that we can find inspiration to do something similar in our own communities.

But there was one statement that I made in the beginning that I have left incomplete until now. This statement may shed some light on what is necessary to help those who hold within their grasp the power to unleash vast resources for global healing find illumination, and help them realize their commonality with the rest of humanity.

I stated that we must embody Ayurveda.

What does that mean?

To me, this is a fundamental question, that asks: what lies within the deepest recesses of our hearts waiting to blossom? If the Rishis had a prayer for the future of their lineage, what would it be? I suspect that it would be that we would come to know what they knew, to see what they saw, to understand what they understood, to feel what they felt.

In my opinion, Ayurveda has a major role to play in the spiritual awakening of humanity. I would define this simply as an awakening of caring for others, an awakening of sharing, an awakening of love for the earth, an awakening of tolerance for our differences.

I believe Ayurveda can bring about this awakening, individually first and eventually collectively, for this reason: if it is not the only, it is certainly the best, most comprehensive, easily comprehendible, non-sectarian, biologically based system of holistic macrothinking that reveals to humanity its deeper elemental and pranic identity and its inherent interconnectedness with all life, and thereby has the capacity to heal the ancient wound of separation between humans and nature, brain and heart, men and women, wealthy and poor, oppressor and oppressed.

It has the power to do this, because, as I also stated earlier, Ayurveda is the living energetic and elemental reality of our physiology, and therefore accessible to everyone regardless of national, cultural, racial, ethnic or religious habits of the ahamkar.

How can Ayurveda heal these ancient wounds?

By teaching us about agni; if we then contemplate the presence of agni within us, we come to know that agni is inside all other beings as well.

By teaching us about prana; if we then contemplate the presence of prana within us, we come to know that prana is inside all other beings as well.

By teaching us about earth and water and air; if we then contemplate the presence of earth and water and air within us, we come to know that these elements are inside all other beings as well.

All the forms of human goodness that are being expressed by the great Dharmic movements that share solidarity of vision and purpose with Ayurveda, and all the ways we are bringing Ayurveda into the world along with those movements, all rest on one fundamental ability: to feel our interconnectedness to the world. Without that ability, humanity has very little chance of surviving for much longer.

This is what Ayurveda means to me.

Therefore, in closing, I will repeat again my personal definition of Ayurveda: if it is not the only, it is certainly the best, most comprehensive, easily comprehendible, non-sectarian, biologically based system of holistic macrothinking that reveals to humanity its deeper elemental and pranic identity and its inherent interconnectedness with all life.

David Crow is one of the world's foremost experts and leading speakers in the field of botanical medicine and grassroots healthcare. He is a master herbalist, aromatherapist and acupuncturist with over 30 years experience and is an expert in the Ayurvedic and Chinese medical systems. David is the author of *In Search of the Medicine Buddha* and *Sacred Smoke*, and the founder and president of Floracopeia, Inc.

To learn more about David Crow and Floracopeia, Inc. products please visit **www.floracopeia.com**.

Also by David Crow:
In Search of the Medicine Buddha

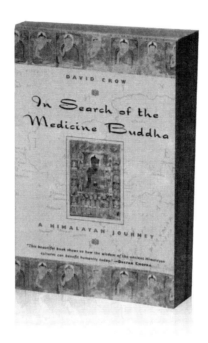

A colorful and captivating story of adventure, exploration, and self discovery, In Search of the Medicine Buddha transports readers into the life and work of David Crow and his teachers of medicine. It is a journey into the wonders of Himalayan herbology and spirituality, written in lyrical prose that interweaves valuable medical teachings with insights into the Buddhist and Hindu cultures of Nepal. Appealing to those interested in exotic places and genuine mystical encounters, this account of one man's search for authentic lineages of Himalayan medicine evokes the beauty and wonder of a faraway land, and reveals a hidden world of powerful and increasingly important healing knowledge.

"David Crow's vision of enlisting the healing plants in the effort to heal the the environment is an excellent insight, really illuminating, and beautiful as well. He writes beautifully and he has a solid knowledge of the plant kingdom and its role in salvaging our health from its currently predicament.

David makes the ancient teachings of Ayurveda, Chinese medicine, and Tibetan medicine relevant to our times, without compromising his respect and reverence for the traditions. I absolutely loved it. So did everyone else I gave a copy to."

Robert Thurman

"This beautiful book shows us how the wisdom of the ancient Himalayan cultures can benefit humanity today."

Deepak Chopra, M.D.
Author of "How to Know God"

"David Crow provides great insights into the healing practices of Tibetan medicine and Buddhism. This book is a wonderful integration of spirituality and medicine."

Dr. Vasant Lad
Author of "Ayuveda: The Science of Self-Healing"

"A fantastic read! This is a contemporary account of one man's journey into the past to learn the ancient secrets of healing. David Crow's book delves deep into the roots of ancient herbal medicine."

Michael Tierra, L.Ac.
Author of "Planetary Herbology"

"As Indian and Tibetan medicine become popular in the West they, like yoga and meditation, are too often stripped of their rich cultural context. David Crow was fortunate to have met outstanding physicians in his travels, and made the most of his fortune by dedicatedly absorbing what they offered him. His fascinating account of apprenticeship and discovery opens a wide window for the reader into the laboratory of true healing art."

Dr. Robert Svoboda
Author of "Ayurveda: Life, Health, and Longevity"